T0227231

Quality Patient Care: Making Evidence-Based, High Value Choices

Editors

MARC SHALABY
EDWARD R. BOLLARD

MEDICAL CLINICS
OF NORTH AMERICA

www.medical.theclinics.com

Consulting Editors
DOUGLAS S. PAAUW
EDWARD R. BOLLARD

September 2016 • Volume 100 • Number 5

ELSEVIER

1600 John F. Kennedy Boulevard • Suite 1800 • Philadelphia, Pennsylvania, 19103-2899

http://www.theclinics.com

MEDICAL CLINICS OF NORTH AMERICA Volume 100, Number 5
September 2016 ISSN 0025-7125, ISBN-13: 978-0-323-46260-0

Editor: Jessica McCool
Developmental Editor: Alison Swety

© **2016 Elsevier Inc. All rights reserved.**

This periodical and the individual contributions contained in it are protected under copyright by Elsevier, and the following terms and conditions apply to their use:

Photocopying
Single photocopies of single articles may be made for personal use as allowed by national copyright laws. Permission of the Publisher and payment of a fee is required for all other photocopying, including multiple or systematic copying, copying for advertising or promotional purposes, resale, and all forms of document delivery. Special rates are available for educational institutions that wish to make photocopies for non-profit educational classroom use. For information on how to seek permission visit www.elsevier.com/permissions or call: (+44) 1865 843830 (UK)/(+1) 215 239 3804 (USA).

Derivative Works
Subscribers may reproduce tables of contents or prepare lists of articles including abstracts for internal circulation within their institutions. Permission of the Publisher is required for resale or distribution outside the institution. Permission of the Publisher is required for all other derivative works, including compilations and translations (please consult www.elsevier.com/permissions).

Electronic Storage or Usage
Permission of the Publisher is required to store or use electronically any material contained in this periodical, including any article or part of an article (please consult www.elsevier.com/permissions). Except as outlined above, no part of this publication may be reproduced, stored in a retrieval system or transmitted in any form or by any means, electronic, mechanical, photocopying, recording or otherwise, without prior written permission of the Publisher.

Notice
No responsibility is assumed by the Publisher for any injury and/or damage to persons or property as a matter of products liability, negligence or otherwise, or from any use or operation of any methods, products, instructions or ideas contained in the material herein. Because of rapid advances in the medical sciences, in particular, independent verification of diagnoses and drug dosages should be made.

Although all advertising material is expected to conform to ethical (medical) standards, inclusion in this publication does not constitute a guarantee or endorsement of the quality or value of such product or of the claims made of it by its manufacturer.

Medical Clinics of North America (ISSN 0025-7125) is published bimonthly by Elsevier Inc., 360 Park Avenue South, New York, NY 10010-1710. Months of publication are January, March, May, July, September, and November. Business and editorial offices: 1600 John F. Kennedy Boulevard, Suite 1800, Philadelphia, PA 19103-2899. Periodicals postage paid at New York, NY, and additional mailing offices. Subscription prices are USD $260.00 per year (US individuals), $531.00 per year (US institutions), $100.00 per year (US Students), $320.00 per year (Canadian individuals), $690.00 per year (Canadian institutions), $200.00 per year (Canadian and foreign students), $390.00 per year (foreign individuals), and $690.00 per year (foreign institutions). To receive student/resident rate, orders must be accompanied by name of affiliated institution, date of term, and the signature of program/residency coordinator on institution letterhead. Orders will be billed at individual rate until proof of status is received. Foreign air speed delivery is included in all Clinics' subscription prices. All prices are subject to change without notice. **POSTMASTER:** Send address changes to *Medical Clinics of North America*, Elsevier Health Sciences Division, Subscription Customer Service, 3251 Riverport Lane, Maryland Heights, MO 63043. **Customer Service: Telephone: 1-800-654-2452** (U.S. and Canada); **1-314-447-8871** (outside U.S. and Canada). **Fax: 314-447-8029. E-mail: journalscustomerserviceusa@elsevier.com** (for print support); **journalsonlinesupport-usa@elsevier.com** (for online support).

Reprints. For copies of 100 or more of articles in this publication, please contact the Commercial Reprints Department, Elsevier Inc., 360 Park Avenue South, New York, NY 10010-1710. Tel.: 212-633-3874; Fax: 212-633-3820; E-mail: reprints@elsevier.com.

Medical Clinics of North America is also published in Spanish by McGraw-Hill Interamericana Editores S. A., P.O. Box 5-237, 06500 Mexico, D.F., Mexico.

Medical Clinics of North America is covered in *MEDLINE/PubMed (Index Medicus), Current Contents, ASCA, Excerpta Medica, Science Citation Index,* and *ISI/BIOMED.*

PROGRAM OBJECTIVE
The goal of the *Medical Clinics of North America* is to keep practicing physicians up to date with current clinical practice by providing timely articles reviewing the state of the art in patient care.

TARGET AUDIENCE
All practicing physicians and other healthcare professionals.

LEARNING OBJECTIVES
Upon completion of this activity, participants will be able to:
1. Review cost-effective evaluation of headaches and syncope.
2. Discuss evidence-based evaluations of complaints such as chronic cough and palpitations.
3. Recognize the best therapies and screening methods to optimize patient care and evidence-based practice.

ACCREDITATION
The Elsevier Office of Continuing Medical Education (EOCME) is accredited by the Accreditation Council for Continuing Medical Education (ACCME) to provide continuing medical education for physicians.

The EOCME designates this enduring material for a maximum of 15 *AMA PRA Category 1 Credit*(s)™. Physicians should claim only the credit commensurate with the extent of their participation in the activity.

All other health care professionals requesting continuing education credit for this enduring material will be issued a certificate of participation.

DISCLOSURE OF CONFLICTS OF INTEREST
The EOCME assesses conflict of interest with its instructors, faculty, planners, and other individuals who are in a position to control the content of CME activities. All relevant conflicts of interest that are identified are thoroughly vetted by EOCME for fair balance, scientific objectivity, and patient care recommendations. EOCME is committed to providing its learners with CME activities that promote improvements or quality in healthcare and not a specific proprietary business or a commercial interest.

The planning committee, staff, authors and editors listed below have identified no financial relationships or relationships to products or devices they or their spouse/life partner have with commercial interest related to the content of this CME activity:

Andreas Achilleos, MD, FACP; David J. Aizenberg, MD; Steven Angus, MD, FACP; Jennifer Baldwin, MD; Edward R. Bollard, MD, DDS, FACP; Robert K. Cato, MD; Jaclyn Cox, DO, FACP; Anjali Fortna; Eliana V. Hempel, MD; Marilyn Katz, MD, FACP; Margaret Kreher, MD; Meghan E. Lembeck, MD; Allison Magnuson, DO; Jessica McCool; Premkumar Nandhakumar; Edgar R. Naut, MD; Kerri Palamara, MD; Colette R. Pameijer, MD; Padmanabhan Premkumar, MD; Matthew H. Rusk, MD; Marissa C. Salvo, PharmD, BCACP; Marc Shalaby, MD, FACP; Ashley H. Snyder, MD; Megan Suermann; Ruchir Trivedi, MD, MMedSci, MRCP(UK); Amy M. Westcott, MD; Joel Wilken, DO.

UNAPPROVED/OFF-LABEL USE DISCLOSURE
The EOCME requires CME faculty to disclose to the participants:
1. When products or procedures being discussed are off-label, unlabelled, experimental, and/or investigational (not US Food and Drug Administration [FDA] approved); and
2. Any limitations on the information presented, such as data that are preliminary or that represent ongoing research, interim analyses, and/or unsupported opinions. Faculty may discuss information about pharmaceutical agents that is outside of FDA-approved labelling. This information is intended solely for CME and is not intended to promote off-label use of these medications. If you have any questions, contact the medical affairs department of the manufacturer for the most recent prescribing information.

TO ENROLL
To enroll in the *Medical Clinics of North America* Continuing Medical Education program, call customer service at 1-800-654-2452 or sign up online at http://www.theclinics.com/home/cme. The CME program is available to subscribers for an additional annual fee of USD $295.

METHOD OF PARTICIPATION
In order to claim credit, participants must complete the following:
1. Complete enrolment as indicated above.
2. Read the activity.

3. Complete the CME Test and Evaluation. Participants must achieve a score of 70% on the test. All CME Tests and Evaluations must be completed online.

CME INQUIRIES/SPECIAL NEEDS

For all CME inquiries or special needs, please contact elsevierCME@elsevier.com.

MEDICAL CLINICS OF NORTH AMERICA

RELATED INTEREST

Nursing Clinics of North America, March 2015 (Vol. 50, Issue 1)
Transformational Tool Kit for Front Line Nurses
Francisca Cisneros Farrar, *Editor*
http://www.nursing.theclinics.com/

THE CLINICS ARE AVAILABLE ONLINE!
Access your subscription at:
www.theclinics.com

Contributors

CONSULTING EDITORS

DOUGLAS S. PAAUW, MD, MACP
Professor of Medicine, Division of General Internal Medicine, Rathmann Family Foundation Endowed Chair for Patient-Centered Clinical Education; Medicine Student Programs, Professor of Medicine, University of Washington School of Medicine, Seattle, Washington

EDWARD R. BOLLARD, MD, DDS, FACP
Professor of Medicine, Associate Dean of Graduate Medical Education, Designated Institutional Official, Department of Medicine, Penn State-Hershey Medical Center, Penn State University College of Medicine, Hershey, Pennsylvania

EDITORS

MARC SHALABY, MD, FACP
Program Director, Internal Medicine-Primary Care Residency, Associate Professor of Clinical Medicine, Perelman School of Medicine at the University of Pennsylvania, Philadelphia, Pennsylvania

EDWARD R. BOLLARD, MD, DDS, FACP
Professor of Medicine, Associate Dean of Graduate Medical Education, Designated Institutional Official, Department of Medicine, Penn State-Hershey Medical Center, Penn State University College of Medicine, Hershey, Pennsylvania

AUTHORS

ANDREAS ACHILLEOS, MD, FACP
Assistant Professor; Associate Program Director; Internal Medicine Residency Program, Internal Medicine, Penn State-Hershey Medical Center, Hershey, Pennsylvania

DAVID J. AIZENBERG, MD
Assistant Professor of Clinical Medicine, Perelman School of Medicine at the University of Pennsylvania, Philadelphia, Pennsylvania

STEVEN ANGUS, MD, FACP
Program Director and Vice-Chair of Education, Associate Professor, Department of Medicine, University of Connecticut School of Medicine, Farmington, Connecticut

JENNIFER BALDWIN, MD
Associate Program Director, Internal Medicine Residency, University of Connecticut, Farmington, Connecticut

EDWARD R. BOLLARD, MD, DDS, FACP
Professor of Medicine, Associate Dean of Graduate Medical Education, Designated Institutional Official, Department of Medicine, Penn State-Hershey Medical Center, Penn State University College of Medicine, Hershey, Pennsylvania

ROBERT K. CATO, MD
Professor of Clinical Medicine, Division of General Internal Medicine, Penn Center for Primary Care, Perelman School of Medicine at the University of Pennsylvania, Philadelphia, Pennsylvania

JACLYN COX, DO, FACP
Osteopathic Tract Director, Internal Medicine Residency, University of Connecticut, Farmington, Connecticut

ELIANA V. HEMPEL, MD
Assistant Professor, Department of Medicine, Penn State-Hershey Medical Center, Hershey, Pennsylvania

MARILYN KATZ, MD, FACP
Assistant Professor of Medicine, University of Connecticut School of Medicine, Farmington, Connecticut

MARGARET KREHER, MD
Associate Professor, Department of Medicine, Center of Excellence in Palliative Medicine, Palliative Care, Penn State-Hershey Medical Center, Hershey, Pennsylvania

MEGHAN E. LEMBECK, MD
Attending Physician; Internal Medicine, PinnacleHealth Primary Care, Annville Family Medicine, Annville, Pennsylvania

ALLISON MAGNUSON, DO
Senior Instructor, Division of Hematology/Oncology, Wilmot Cancer Institute, University of Rochester, Rochester, New York

EDGAR R. NAUT, MD
Assistant Professor of Medicine, University of Connecticut, Saint Francis Hospital and Medical Center, Hartford, Connecticut

KERRI PALAMARA, MD
Assistant Professor, Harvard Medical School, Boston, Massachusetts

COLETTE R. PAMEIJER, MD
Associate Professor; General Surgical Specialties & Surgical Oncology, Penn State University College of Medicine, Hershey, Pennsylvania

PADMANABHAN PREMKUMAR, MD
Assistant Professor of Medicine, UCONN Health; Site Director, Internal Medicine Training Program, UCONN Health/Hartford Hospital, Hartford, Connecticut

MATTHEW H. RUSK, MD
Professor of Clinical Medicine, Division of General Internal Medicine, Perelman School of Medicine at the University of Pennsylvania, Philadelphia, Pennsylvania

MARISSA C. SALVO, PharmD, BCACP
Assistant Clinical Professor, Department of Pharmacy Practice, University of Connecticut School of Pharmacy, Storrs, Connecticut

ASHLEY H. SNYDER, MD
Fellow, Division of General Internal Medicine, Penn State-Hershey Medical Center, Hershey, Pennsylvania

RUCHIR TRIVEDI, MD, MMedSci, MRCP(UK)
Assistant Professor, Division of Nephrology, Department of Medicine, University of Connecticut, Farmington, Connecticut

AMY M. WESTCOTT, MD
Associate Professor, Geriatric and Palliative Medicine, Department of Medicine, Penn State-Hershey Medical Center, Penn State University College of Medicine, Hershey, Pennsylvania

JOEL WILKEN, DO
Assistant Director, Ambulatory Site Director, Department of Medicine, Hartford Hospital, Hartford, Connecticut; Assistant Professor, University of Connecticut, School of Medicine, Farmington, Connecticut

Contents

> Approximately one-third of deaths in the United States are from cardiovascular disease. Managing modifiable risk factors is paramount to reducing risk of heart disease and stroke. It is logical to try to identify patients with silent disease that may predispose them to significant morbidity and mortality. Unfortunately, it is unclear if routine screening for the presence of carotid stenosis, coronary artery disease, and peripheral arterial disease is beneficial. Many of these tests are expensive. This review explores the evidence behind screening tests, costs associated with the tests, and the implications of positive screening for each of the 3 listed conditions.

> Palpitations are a symptom of many cardiac and noncardiac conditions. The patient's history, physical examination, appropriately directed laboratory tests, and basic electrocardiogram are helpful in evaluating palpitations and may be essential to finding a diagnosis. There are many outpatient options for the evaluation of palpitations caused by a presumed cardiogenic cause. These evaluation tools include Holter monitor, event monitor, transtelephonic electrocardiographic monitor, treadmill exercise stress test, echocardiography, and electrophysiologic studies. Most patients can be evaluated as an outpatient, but there are reasons, such as hemodynamic compromise, that may require admission to an inpatient setting to complete the diagnostic workup.

> Valvular heart disease is a common condition in today's patient population. Accurate characterization of vital cardiac structures has become crucial to early diagnosis and varied treatment options. The advent of ultrasound technology has had a large impact in cardiovascular medicine, particularly in the assessment of valvular heart disease. Today its versatility and availability have allowed it to become one of the most frequently ordered imaging tests for cardiovascular indications. Despite the tremendous evidence that suggests that clinical examinations are still standard of care, a large volume of referrals for echocardiograms suggests differently.

Occult gastrointestinal bleeding is not visible and may present with a positive fecal occult blood test or iron deficiency anemia. Obscure bleeding can be overt or occult, with no source identified despite an appropriate diagnostic workup. A stepwise approach to this evaluation after negative upper and lower endoscopy has been shown to be cost effective. This includes repeat endoscopies if warranted, followed by video capsule endoscopy (VCE) if no obstruction is present. If the VCE is positive then specific endoscopic intervention may be possible. If negative, patients may undergo either repeat testing or watchful waiting with iron supplements.

Approximately 10% to 15% of patients who experience chronic gastroesophageal reflux disease have Barrett esophagus, which is associated with an increased risk of esophageal adenocarcinoma. If symptoms persist after 8 weeks of adhering to treatment and lifestyle modifications, or if alarm symptoms develop, patients should be referred for screening upper endoscopy. Those with evidence of Barrett esophagus with dysplasia should be monitored in an endoscopic surveillance program, and those with high-grade dysplasia should consider surgical treatment.

Anemia is a prevalent disease with multiple possible etiologies and resultant complications. Iron deficiency anemia is a common cause of anemia and is typically due to insufficient intake, poor absorption, or overt or occult blood loss. Distinguishing iron deficiency from other causes of anemia is integral to initiating the appropriate treatment. In addition, identifying the underlying cause of iron deficiency is also necessary to help guide management of these patients. We review the key components to an evidence-based, cost-conscious evaluation of suspected iron deficiency anemia.

Pain related to various musculoskeletal conditions is a common patient complaint, and one that is often difficult to remedy. In addition to oral analgesics and physical therapy, local injections (most commonly of corticosteroids) are a common intervention and have been for decades. However, in most cases, the literature is full of poor-quality studies, making the true utility of these injections questionable. This article reviews some of the literature studying these injections with the goal of providing clinicians the information to make evidence-based, high-value choices.

effective and less costly than oxygen therapy. Further research is needed in the assessment and treatment of this symptom to more effectively treat patients.

Preface

A Convergence of Themes: Making Evidence-Based, High Value Choices

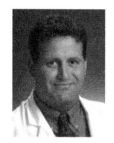 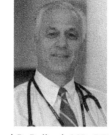

Marc Shalaby, MD, FACP   Edward R. Bollard, MD, DDS, FACP
Editors

It would probably not be accurate to say that medicine is undergoing a revolution. It is more likely that the idea of "revolution" has been repeatedly applied to what has been evolving in health care in each of the last 50 years. We believe it is more accurate to state that each generation of physicians faces its own struggles, its own challenges, and its own opportunities and strives to implement its own innovations. In addition, each generation of physicians has nostalgic notions of what medicine used to be and anxiety about what medicine should and will be in the future.

Over the past 20 years, there has been an increased reliance and respect for evidence-based medicine, quality improvement, population health, using data to drive clinical changes, efficiency and effectiveness, and high-value care. In addition, there has been an outcry for patient centeredness, patient safety, shared decision making, and the importance of the provider/patient relationship.

Given this multitude of interests and themes, each with its own tag name, many physicians have grown weary of the "next thing." In an effort to keep up with these evolving trends, many health systems have adopted short-term, sometimes shortsighted, incentives for the latest "trends." This has often occurred at the expense of practicing clinicians, who have been bludgeoned by electronic health records, quality metrics, pay for performance, and whatever "theme du jour" that happens to be invoked for that particular timeframe.

As physicians who have witnessed massive changes over the last several decades, we now see that we are not merely on the precipice of the "latest and greatest" in health care, but rather at a convergence of the themes that have most recently dominated the improvement of health care. We see that all of these themes—managed care, evidence-based medicine, patient-centered care, quality and system improvement, shared decision making, bending the cost curve, and population health—are

Med Clin N Am 100 (2016) xvii–xviii
http://dx.doi.org/10.1016/j.mcna.2016.06.013
0025-7125/16/$ – see front matter © 2016 Published by Elsevier Inc.

medical.theclinics.com

being applied as we conceptualize what health care will look like in the coming decades. While all of these trends have appeared to be seemingly unrelated, they have been converging and driving toward the same goal: increasingly higher-quality, safer health care for the most people at the least cost.

We are now being called on to engage with our patients on a personal and population level. We need to make decisions about health care that have been proven to be effective and to avoid those tests, medicines, and procedures that have been shown unequivocally not to have value. We must educate our patients so we may engage in a conversation of what is necessary and what is not. We must be stewards of population health care as we provide care for each individual patient.

The purpose of this issue of *Medical Clinics of North America* on "Quality Patient Care: Making Evidence-Based, High Value Choices" is to help inform clinicians about common medical conditions encountered in their practices and provide insight into making better diagnostic and treatment choices as we move toward more effective, more efficient, high-value care.

Marc Shalaby, MD, FACP
Perelman School of Medicine
at the University of Pennsylvania
Penn Center for Primary Care
51 North 39th Street
Medical Arts Building Suite 102
Philadelphia, PA 19104, USA

Edward R. Bollard, MD, DDS, FACP
Penn State-Hershey Medical Center
Penn State University College of Medicine
500 University Drive
Hershey, PA 17033, USA

E-mail addresses:
Marc.Shalaby@uphs.upenn.edu (M. Shalaby)
ebollard@hmc.psu.edu (E.R. Bollard)

Cardiovascular Testing in Asymptomatic Patients

Carotid Duplex, Cardiac Stress Testing, Screen for Peripheral Arterial Disease

David J. Aizenberg, MD

KEYWORDS

- Cardiovascular screening • Carotid artery stenosis • Peripheral vascular disease
- Cardiac stress testing

KEY POINTS

- Screening patients who are at high risk for asymptomatic carotid artery stenosis is unnecessary because they should already be on intense medical therapy and revascularization is unlikely to benefit them.
- Do not perform cardiac stress testing in asymptomatic, low-risk individuals.
- Only perform cardiac stress testing in asymptomatic patients if it will change medication management decisions.
- Revascularization procedures in patients with asymptomatic peripheral arterial disease do not improve outcomes.

INTRODUCTION

Approximately one-third of all deaths in the United States are from cardiovascular disease.[1,2] Managing modifiable risk factors, such as smoking, hypertension, and hyperlipidemia, is paramount to reducing an individual's risk of heart disease and stroke. It is logical to try to identify patients with silent disease that may predispose them to significant morbidity and mortality. Unfortunately, it is unclear if routine screening for the presence of carotid stenosis, coronary artery disease (CAD), and peripheral arterial disease is beneficial. Many of these tests, especially cardiac stress tests, are financially costly. This review explores the evidence behind screening tests, costs associated with the tests, and the implications of positive screening for each of the 3 listed conditions.

Department of Medicine, Perelman School of Medicine, University of Pennsylvania, 3701 Market Street, 7th Floor, Philadelphia, PA 19104, USA
E-mail address: David.aizenberg@uphs.upenn.edu

Med Clin N Am 100 (2016) 971–979
http://dx.doi.org/10.1016/j.mcna.2016.04.004
0025-7125/16/$ – see front matter
© 2016 Elsevier Inc. All rights reserved.

CAROTID DUPLEX
The Disease

Carotid artery stenosis is the narrowing of the internal and/or the common carotid artery by atherosclerosis. It is frequently asymptomatic. The measurement of stenosis depends on the method being used but is commonly reported as the percentage reduction of the luminal diameter. Furthermore, studies vary in how they define moderate or severe stenosis. The most feared complication of carotid artery stenosis is an ischemic stroke. Stroke is the leading cause of serious long-term disability in this country.[2]

The prevalence of carotid artery stenosis in the general population increases with age. A 2010 meta-analysis found that in patients ≤50 years old, the prevalence of severe stenosis (defined as ≥70%) is very low (0.1% in men and 0% in women). This increases with age to 3.1% in men ≥80 years of age and 0.9% in woman of the same age.[3] Approximately 800,000 people in the United States suffer a stroke each year. It is estimated that 90% of all strokes in the United States are ischemic and 10% of ischemic strokes are caused by carotid artery stenosis.[4]

Possible Interventions

It is well established that most patients with *symptomatic* carotid artery stenosis (transient ischemic attack or stroke) should undergo vascular intervention[5] in addition to optimizing medical management with antiplatelet agents, statins, and antihypertensives. This has been shown to reduce the incidence of future cerebrovascular events. These same options are available for individuals with asymptomatic carotid artery stenosis, including carotid endarterectomy, carotid artery stenting, and intensification of medical management, but it is unclear if this would provide the same benefit.

Test Characteristics

The most frequently used modality for detecting carotid artery stenosis is the carotid duplex: an ultrasound test that is painless and does not pose any risk to the patient (from the test alone). The sensitivity and specificity for this test depends on the degree of stenosis that one is looking for. One meta-analysis reported a sensitivity of 90% and a specificity of 94% in detecting a stenosis ≥70%.[6] These values are consistent with other studies evaluating similar degrees of stenosis. It is important to note that clinically relevant variability in performing and interpreting these studies exists and has been reported.[7]

The financial cost of carotid duplex studies is not insignificant. Healthcare Bluebook estimates the average fair price is $388 per study.[8] Patients identified as having mild to moderate carotid artery stenosis may then go on to annual testing for progression. After only 3 years, the cost of this strategy exceeds $1000.

Potential Benefits

The goal of screening asymptomatic patients for carotid artery stenosis is to identify patients at higher risk for stroke and to alter the management in these patients to reduce this risk. In addition to reducing the risk of stroke, patients identified as having carotid artery stenosis may also benefit by being placed in higher risk categories for CAD, and intensifying medical management. This may reduce these individuals' risk of cardiovascular events in the future.

There have been several trials that have demonstrated the utility of carotid endarterectomy for patients with asymptomatic severe carotid stenosis. A Cochrane review of this topic found that this intervention reduced the risk of stroke by 30% over 3 years but that the absolute risk reduction was only 1%.[9] It is important to note that the trials in this review were done without standardization of medical management and before the relatively widespread use of statin therapy. Recent studies find that patients with asymptomatic carotid stenosis who are treated with optimal medical therapy (hypertension management, antiplatelet agents, and statins) have an approximate risk of stroke of 1% per year.[10,11] Even with advancement in surgical techniques, carotid endarterectomy is associated with an estimated perioperative risk of stroke or death of 1.2%.[12] Although there may be some very high-risk patients who would benefit from surgical intervention, there is no evidence that optimal medical therapy is inferior to revascularization.[11]

Potential Harms

As in any screening test, the potential harms of a screening test include those associated with false-positive tests (anxiety, unnecessary testing) and those associated with downstream testing and intervention. A positive carotid duplex is usually followed by carotid angiography. This is an invasive procedure with inherent risks. It requires the insertion of a catheter, the use of contrast, and exposure to radiation. In addition, there is a not-insignificant risk of stroke (up to 1.2%) during the diagnostic angiography.[4] Finally, patients undergoing carotid endarterectomy for asymptomatic carotid stenosis face potential surgical complications, including stroke, perioperative myocardial infarctions, infections, and nerve damage. The meta-analysis performed for the US Preventive Services Task Force (USPSTF) found that 1.9% more participants treated with endarterectomy experienced stroke or death when compared with medical management alone.[4] Furthermore, incidental findings may lead to additional costly and perhaps unnecessary tests. For example, incidental thyroid abnormalities can be found in more than 20% of patients undergoing carotid ultrasound.[13]

Guidelines

Most professional societies have moved away, or are moving away, from recommending screening for carotid artery stenosis. In 2011, The American Heart Association (AHA) and the American Stroke Association (ASA) issued extensive guidelines for the primary prevention of stroke.[10] They note that medical therapy has significantly changed since the clinical trials that showed a benefit to surgical intervention, and that there is now uncertainty whether to recommend surgery in asymptomatic patients. In those guidelines, they do not recommend screening in the general population for asymptomatic carotid stenosis. In that same year (2011), the AHA, ASA, and 12 other groups issued a joint statement of guidelines that stated that carotid duplex screening is not recommended for routine screening in asymptomatic patients who have no clinical manifestations of or risk factors for atherosclerosis.[14] They do state that it is reasonable to screen those with symptomatic CAD or peripheral vascular disease, but it is unclear if a positive screen would change those patients' management. As of July 2014, the USPSTF gives screening for asymptomatic carotid stenosis a "D" recommendation, meaning that there is a "moderate or high certainty that the service has no net benefit or that the harms outweigh the benefits."[4]

Summary

Asymptomatic carotid artery stenosis has low prevalence in the general population. Although the carotid duplex has relatively favorable test characteristics, routine screening for a low prevalence finding will lead to a substantial number of false positives and downstream unnecessary consequences. Furthermore, it is unclear if surgical management of this disease offers any additional benefit to intensive medical therapy alone. Therefore, it seems that it would be beneficial to screen patients only if an intensification of medications is an option. Most societies recommend against screening the general population for carotid artery stenosis. Some advocate the use of carotid artery duplex to screen patients at higher risk, but it is unclear if identifying these patients would alter their management because they should already be on intensive medical therapy.

CARDIAC STRESS TESTING
The Disease

In 2015, the AHA reported that 15.5 million American adults have coronary heart disease.[2] This includes 7.6 million with myocardial infarctions, and 8.2 million with angina pectoris. Heart disease is the leading cause of death in the United States, accounting for more than 600,000 deaths per year.[1] Most of these deaths are from myocardial infarction, a direct result of atherosclerosis of the coronary arteries. With advances in medical and interventional therapies, death rates attributable to cardiovascular disease have declined since 2000.[2]

Silent ischemia is defined as objective evidence of myocardial ischemia in patients without symptoms.[15] This could occur in patients with known stable CAD or in patients who have no history of CAD. For the purposes of this review, we limit the scope to patients without known CAD.

The prevalence of asymptomatic coronary heart disease and silent ischemia varies widely depending on patients' risk factors. Diabetes mellitus is a major risk factor that increases the likelihood of having silent ischemia. One meta-analysis found an adjusted hazard ratio of 2.0 for CAD in asymptomatic patients with diabetes. Stress testing is positive in approximately 20% of asymptomatic patients with diabetes.[16]

Possible Interventions

Identification of silent myocardial ischemia could potentially lead to further diagnostic tests and interventions. Unlike symptomatic angina pectoris, intervening on silent ischemia, by definition, does not alter symptoms. Any change in management is geared toward improving future outcomes. If asymptomatic coronary heart disease is detected, possible interventions include intensifying medical management (eg, antiplatelet agents, beta-blockers, and statin therapy) or revascularization (eg, percutaneous coronary intervention or coronary artery bypass grafting).

Test Characteristics

Silent myocardial ischemia in patients without a known history of CAD is most commonly diagnosed by stress testing; either exercise testing alone (with electrocardiogram [ECG]) or in combination with nuclear or echocardiogram imaging.[15,17] In one meta-analysis, the sensitivity and specificity of exercise ECG testing varied widely.[18] The mean sensitivity was 68% and the mean specificity was 77%. This variability was again demonstrated in an analysis of data from a multicenter trial of 2800 asymptomatic individuals undergoing exercise testing.[19] The standard deviation of sensitivity and specificity reported there were 13% and 5%, respectively. Exercise ECG testing has been shown to contribute to prognostic information. In the Multiple Risk Factor Intervention Trial (MRFIT), more than 12,000 men without known CAD, but a high risk of future events (history of smoking, elevated cholesterol, or elevated diastolic blood pressure) were screened with exercise ECG testing.[20] In this trial, there was almost a fourfold increase in 7-year coronary mortality in those men with an abnormal response to exercise.

With regard to stress testing with imaging (eg, radionucleotide myocardial perfusion or echocardiogram), the sensitivity is higher (70%–90%) but the specificity is the same as exercise ECG stress.[21] The addition of an imaging technique does help quantify the area of ischemia and the size of the defect.[22]

The Healthcare Bluebook estimates the average fair price for cardiac perfusion imaging to be $1078.[13] This is the most expensive testing modality. As a comparison, the estimated fair price for an exercise ECG stress test is $147.

Potential Benefits

If asymptomatic CAD or silent ischemia is diagnosed, then the potential benefits of intervention are to reduce future events, including death. Medically managing asymptomatic CAD would also likely reduce the risk of cerebrovascular events. In addition, from a patient's point of view, being labeled as having a "heart condition" may provide additional motivation to adhere to recommended treatments or lifestyle modification.

Potential Harms

The BARDOT trial evaluated 400 asymptomatic patients with type 2 diabetes who were on optimal medical therapy. Consistent with other trials, 22% of these patients had a positive radionucleotide myocardial perfusion imaging. Patients with a positive stress test were then randomized to medical therapy alone (39 patients) or to an invasive revascularization intervention group (43 patients). Overall, the number of events in this study was low. Two deaths (4.7%) in the medical therapy group were attributed to a cardiac etiology compared with 0 in the revascularization group. Six patients (15.4%) in the medical therapy group had major adverse cardiac events compared with 2 patients (4.7%) in the revascularization group. It is important to note that none of these differences were statistically significant.[23] Identifying patients with silent ischemia may start a patient on the path to more invasive testing and intervention, such as left heart catheterization with percutaneous coronary intervention. This predisposes patients to harms, such as bleeding, vascular injury, and in-stent thrombosis.

Guidelines

All major guidelines recommend against screening low-risk asymptomatic patients for coronary heart disease. There is some disagreement about what to do with patients who are at higher risk. In 2002, the American College of Cardiology and the AHA identified some groups that may benefit from screening for asymptomatic CAD.[24] Such patients include those with diabetes mellitus who are about to begin a vigorous exercise program, patients with multiple risk factors who are not on intensive medical therapy, asymptomatic patients (men >45 years, women >55 years) who plan to start vigorous exercise (especially if sedentary), or those in which impairment might impact public safety. The USPSTF concluded in 2012 that there were insufficient data to recommend for or against the use of resting or exercise ECGs in patients at intermediate or high risk for CAD.[25]

Summary

Screening cardiac stress testing in low-risk individuals who are asymptomatic is not indicated. In those who are at higher risk because of various risk factors, including diabetes, smoking, hypertension, and family history, screening could be considered if medication management will be altered with a positive test. Revascularization of asymptomatic patients without a history of CAD is not recommend and should not be a reason to perform cardiac stress testing.

SCREEN FOR PERIPHERAL ARTERIAL DISEASE
The Disease

Peripheral arterial disease (PAD) is atherosclerotic occlusion of arteries outside of the heart. Risk factors associated with PAD are similar to those associated with CAD (smoking, hypertension, hypercholesterolemia, and diabetes).[26] PAD prevalence is low in persons younger than 50 and increases with age in both men and women. In men, the prevalence is at least 20% by the age of 80. African American individuals have a strikingly higher prevalence of PAD (up to 2 times that of non-Hispanic white Americans).[27] Most patients with PAD and their physicians are unaware of their diagnosis.[28] The classic symptom of PAD is intermittent claudication (pain in the lower extremities with walking that is relieved with rest). The presence of PAD is an independent risk factor for coronary events and all-cause mortality. The presence of PAD doubles the relative risk of death over a 10-year period.[27]

Possible Interventions

Once PAD is diagnosed, medications can be intensified (antiplatelet agents and statins), counseling can be emphasized toward quitting smoking and increasing physical activity, or revascularization can be performed (percutaneous interventions vs bypass grafting).

Test Characteristics

The standard way to screen for or diagnose PAD is by obtaining the ankle-brachial index (ABI). This test uses Doppler to assess the ratio of systolic pressures in the lower extremities to those of the upper extremities. An ABI ≤ 0.9 is considered a positive test. There is little evidence on the test characteristics when used to screen the general population. When evaluating patients with risk factors or suspected PAD, the sensitivity is estimated to be 80% and the specificity to be 97%.[27] Because this is a noninvasive test, there is no harm from the test itself to the patient.

Potential Benefits

Identification of asymptomatic PAD may lead to decreased progression of PAD (increasing symptoms and limb ischemia) through medication adjustment or vascular intervention. Furthermore, diagnosing a patient with PAD may lead to adjustment of management that reduces the risk of other outcomes, such as myocardial infarction and stroke. With regard to medication management, it is unclear if the benefits of aspirin outweigh the harms in asymptomatic patients without CAD. In one study, 3350 patients with low ABI and no evidence of CAD were randomized to receive 100 mg aspirin versus placebo. After a mean follow-up of 8.2 years, there was no difference in mortality or vascular events.[29] It is also unclear if identification of patients with PAD would lead to better adherence to medications, smoking cessation, and increased physical activity.

Potential Harms

Without a clear benefit to identifying patients as having PAD, any intervention may have potential harms. This includes the addition of aspirin, an intervention known to increase the risk of hemorrhage.

Guidelines

There is no clear consensus to guide the decision to screen asymptomatic patients for PAD. In 2011, the American College of Cardiology (ACC) and AHA Task Force on Practice Guidelines recommended screening for ABI in high-risk groups that included all patients older than 65, or those older than 50 who have a history of smoking or diabetes.[30] In 2013, the USPSTF concluded that the current evidence is insufficient to assess the balance of benefits and harms of screening for PAD and cardiovascular disease risk assessment with the ABI in adults.[31]

Summary

The presence of PAD is a marker for an increased risk of cardiovascular events and mortality. Many patients with PAD are asymptomatic. Revascularization procedures do not seem to improve outcomes in asymptomatic patients. It is unclear if patients identified as having PAD benefit from intensification of pharmacologic therapy. Therefore, there is insufficient evidence to recommend for or against screening for PAD.

SUMMARY

Routine screening for asymptomatic cardiovascular disease, such as carotid artery stenosis, CAD, and PAD is costly and exposes patients to unnecessary risks. Patients who have the highest prevalence of these diseases have risk factors that could easily be identified without the costs and harms associated with screening tests. In these patients, even a positive screening test does not inform management decisions because optimal medical management should be already indicated. In all 3 disease processes addressed by this article, optimal medical management is a reasonable and noninferior strategy to reduce the risk of progression and adverse outcomes. Ordering screening tests on patients with a low risk-factor profile (and therefore a lower prevalence of cardiovascular disease), subjects them to a significantly increased risk of a false-positive test leading to more costly and potentially harmful downstream diagnostics and interventions. Clinicians should carefully consider these issues when considering these screening tests.

REFERENCES

1. Centers for Disease Control and Prevention. Leading Causes of Death 2015. Available at: http://www.cdc.gov/nchs/fastats/leading-causes-of-death.htm. Accessed January 10, 2016.
2. Mozaffarian D, Benjamin E, Go A, et al. Heart disease and stroke statistics—2015 update a report from the American Heart Association. Circulation 2015;131: e29–322.
3. de Weerd A, Greving J, Hedblad B, et al. Prevalence of asymptomatic carotid artery stenosis in the general population: an individual participant data meta-analysis. Stroke 2010;41:1294–7.
4. Jonas D, Feltner C, Halle R, et al. Screening for asymptomatic carotid artery stenosis: a systematic review and meta-analysis for the U.S. Preventive Services Task Force. Ann Intern Med 2014;161:336–46.
5. Kernan A, Ovbiagele B, Black H, et al. Guidelines for the prevention of stroke in patients with stroke and transient ischemic attack: a guideline for healthcare professionals from the American Heart Association/American Stroke Association. Stroke 2014;45:2160–236.
6. Jahromi A, Cina C, Liu Y, et al. Sensitivity and specificity of color duplex ultrasound measurement in the estimation of internal carotid artery stenosis: a systematic review and meta-analysis. J Vasc Surg 2005;41:962–72.
7. Normahani P, Aslam M, Martin G, et al. Variation in duplex peak systolic velocity measurement in a multi-site vascular service. Perfusion 2015;30:636–42.

8. CAREOperative. The healthcare blue book. Available at: http://healthcareblue book.com. Accessed March 4, 2016.

9. Chambers B, Donnan G. Carotid endarterectomy for asymptomatic carotid stenosis. Cochrane Database Syst Rev 2005;(4):CD001923.

10. Goldstein L, Bushnell C, Adams R, et al. Guidelines for the primary prevention of stroke: a guideline for healthcare professionals from the American Heart Association/American Stroke Association. Stroke 2011;42:517–84.

11. Raman G, Moorthy D, Hadar N, et al. Management strategies for asymptomatic carotid stenosis a systematic review and meta-analysis. Ann Intern Med 2013; 158:676–85.

12. Munster A, Franchini A, Qureshi M, et al. Temporal trends in safety of carotid endarterectomy in asymptomatic patients systemic review. Neurology 2015;85: 365–72.

13. Rad M, Zakavi S, Layegh P, et al. Incidental thyroid abnormalities on carotid color Doppler ultrasound: frequency and clinical significance. J Med Ultrasound 2015; 23:25–8.

14. Brott T, Halperin J, Abbara S, et al. 2011 ASA/ACCF/AHA/AANN/AANS/ACR/ASNR/CNS/SAIP/SCAI/SIR/SNIS/SVM/SVS guideline on the management of patients with extracranial carotid and vertebral artery disease. Circulation 2011; 124:e54–130.

15. Conti C, Bavry A, Petersen J. Silent ischemia: clinical relevance. J Am Coll Cardiol 2012;59:435–41.

16. Wackers F, Young L, Inzucchi S, et al. Detection of silent myocardial ischemia in asymptomatic diabetic subjects: the DIAD study. Diabetes Care 2004;27: 1954–61.

17. Gutterman D. Silent myocardial ischemia. Circ J 2009;73:785–97.

18. Gianrossi R, Detrano R, Mulvihill D, et al. Exercise-induced ST depression in the diagnosis of coronary artery disease. A meta-analysis. Circulation 1989;80:87–98.

19. Detrano R. Variability in the accuracy of the exercise ST-segment in predicting the coronary angiogram: how good can we be? J Electrocardiol 1992;24(Suppl): 54–61.

20. Rautahariu P, Prineas R, Eifler W, et al. Prognostic value of exercise electrocardiogram in men at high risk of future coronary heart disease: Multiple Risk Factor Intervention Trial experience. J Am Coll Cardiol 1986;8:1–10.

21. Fihn S, Gardin J, Abrams J, et al. 2012 ACCF/AHA/ACP/AATS/PCNA/SCAI/STS guideline for the diagnosis and management of patients with stable ischemic heart disease. Circulation 2012;126:e354.

22. Fleischmann K, Hunink M, Kuntz K, et al. Exercise echocardiography or exercise SPECT imaging? A meta-analysis of diagnostic test performance. JAMA 1998; 280:913–20.

23. Wellweger M, Maraun M, Osterhues H, et al. Progression to overt or silent CAD in asymptomatic patients with diabetes mellitus at high coronary risk: main findings of the prospective multicenter BARDOT trial with a pilot randomized treatment substudy. JACC Cardiovasc Imaging 2014;7:1001–10.

24. Gibbons R, Balady G, Bricker J, et al. ACC/AHA 2002 guideline update for exercise testing: summary article. A report of the American College of Cardiology/American Heart Association Task Force on Practice Guidelines (Committee to Update the 1997 Exercise Testing Guidelines). J Am Coll Cardiol 2002;40:1531–40.

25. Chou R, Arora B, Dana T, et al. Screening asymptomatic adults with resting or exercise electrocardiography: a review of the evidence for the U.S. Preventive Services Task Force. Ann Intern Med 2011;155:375–85.

26. Joosten M, Pai J, Bertoia M, et al. Associations between conventional cardiovascular risk factors and risk of peripheral artery disease in men. JAMA 2012;308: 1660–7.
27. Criqui M, Aboyans V. Epidemiology of peripheral artery disease. Circ Res 2015; 116:1509–26.
28. Novo S. Classification, epidemiology, risk factors, and natural history of peripheral arterial disease. Diabetes Obes Metab 2002;4(Suppl 2):s1–6.
29. Fowkes F, Price J, Stewart M, et al. Aspirin for prevention of cardiovascular events in a general population screened for a low ankle brachial index: a randomized controlled trial. JAMA 2010;303:841–8.
30. Rooke T, Hirsch A, Misra S, et al. 2011 ACCF/AHA focused update of the guideline for the management of patients with peripheral artery disease (updating the 2005 guideline): a report of the American College of Cardiology Foundation/American Heart Association Task Force on Practice Guidelines. J Am Coll Cardiol 2011;58:2020–45.
31. Lin J, Olson C, Johnson E, et al. The ankle–brachial index for peripheral artery disease screening and cardiovascular disease prediction among asymptomatic adults: a systematic evidence review for the U.S. Preventive Services Task Force. Ann Intern Med 2013;159:333–41.

Evidence-based Recommendations for the Evaluation of Palpitations in the Primary Care Setting

Joel Wilken, DO[a,b],*

KEYWORDS

- Palpitations • Evaluation • Arrhythmia • Electrocardiographic monitoring

KEY POINTS

- Primary care and emergency medicine providers are often asked to evaluate and diagnose the complaint of palpitations.
- There are many possible causes for this common patient presentation.
- Several diagnostic modalities are available to help evaluate the cause of palpitations.
- Primary care and emergency medicine providers should have an understanding of the possible causes and the judicious use of diagnostic modalities that are currently available to help discern benign versus more serious causes.

INTRODUCTION

Patient History

A 45-year-old woman with no significant past medical history presents to her primary care physician's office with a chief complaint of a 2-month history of episodic palpitations. The symptoms can happen at rest or with exertion. She is bothered by the "fluttering" sensations in her chest, but they usually only last for about 10 to 15 seconds per episode. She mentions that she could have up to 10 episodes over the course of 10 minutes when they do happen. They are not associated with chest pain or shortness of breath. The patient has researched online about palpitations and is concerned that these symptoms could be related to a heart condition. She asks her primary care physician about the evaluation of these symptoms.

This scenario is a common situation that primary care providers will frequently encounter. Heart palpitations are a subjective sensation of feeling one's heartbeat.

Disclosure Statement: The author has nothing to disclose.
[a] Department of Medicine, Hartford Hospital, 80 Seymour Street, Hartford, CT 06102, USA;
[b] University of Connecticut, School of Medicine, 263 Farmington Avenue, CT 06030, USA
* Department of Medicine, Hartford Hospital, 80 Seymour Street, Hartford, CT 06102.
E-mail address: Joel.Wilken@hhchealth.org

Med Clin N Am 100 (2016) 981–989
http://dx.doi.org/10.1016/j.mcna.2016.04.006
0025-7125/16/$ – see front matter © 2016 Elsevier Inc. All rights reserved.

As many as 16% of patients presenting to their primary care provider report palpitations.[1] Palpitation is a word that is derived from the early fifteenth century from middle French—palpitation, and from Latin—palpitationem. It is a noun of action from the past participle stem of palpitare meaning to throb, to flutter, or to quiver.[2] Palpitations are often described as a perceived abnormality of the heartbeat associated with an awareness of heart muscle contractions in the chest. Palpitations can be recognized as both a symptom and a medical diagnosis. Palpitations may be accompanied by a variety of symptoms or perhaps none at all, often making a patient's symptoms vague, nonspecific, and diagnostically challenging.[3]

There are a variety of diagnostic tests that can be used in the evaluation of palpitations. Some are simple (physical examination) and others are more complex (30-day event monitor). Given the frequency in which patients present with this complaint, it is important to develop an effective, cost-conscious approach to evaluation. Although it would be ideal for the evaluation to determine the exact cause of the symptoms, it more commonly serves to distinguish the benign causes from the more dangerous cardiac causes.[3] The goal of this article is to provide the reader with an understanding of the diagnostic tools available in the evaluation of palpitations and help craft a diagnostic strategy that is medically sound and cost-effective.

PATHOPHYSIOLOGY

"Stop and start" or "flip-flop" are some of the ways in which patients will describe the sensation of palpitations. Usually the "stop" is associated with the cardiac pause following the contraction, and the "start" with the subsequent forceful contractions.[4] Palpitations can usually be attributed to 1 of 4 main causes: extracardiac stimulation of the vagus nerve; pronounced sympathetic response as a consequence of an organic medical condition; hyperdynamic circulation; or abnormal heart rhythms. Possible contributors to these causes are listed in **Table 1**.

Normal cardiac conduction involves the spontaneous discharge of an electrical impulse at the sinoatrial node. The electrical impulse depolarizes the atria and then is conducted to the atrioventricular (AV) node. It then propagates by way of the His-Purkinje system to depolarize the ventricles.[4] If there is a disruption anywhere along this pathway, an arrhythmia may be produced.

Table 1
Causes of palpitations

Cause	Possible Contributors
Extracardiac stimulation of the vagus nerve	Elevations of catecholamines and glucocorticoids associated with stress and anxiety
Pronounced sympathetic response as a consequence of an organic medical condition	• Hypoglycemia • Hypoxia • Heart failure
Hyperdynamic circulation	• Valvular incompetence • Thyrotoxicosis • Hypercapnia • Hyperthermia
Abnormal heart rhythms	• Atrial fibrillation • Ectopic beats • Ventricular arrhythmias • Heart block

A differential diagnosis of cardiac causes of palpitations is summarized in **Table 2** with a more complete discussion of Brugada syndrome in **Box 1** and Postural orthostatic tachycardia syndrome in **Box 2**. Cardiac conditions more commonly found in women can be found in **Box 3**.

In the general population, ventricular ectopy is common. The percentages can be broken down as follows: (a) 50% to 55% of people younger than 30 years of age; (b) 64% to 73% of middle-aged men and women; and (c) an even higher percentage of people older than 60 years of age.[5] More specifically, research indicates that men reporting regular palpitations, individuals experiencing palpitations at work, and those experiencing palpitations during sleep were more likely to have a cardiac cause for their palpitations.[6]

In addition, many noncardiac conditions may also result in palpitations. **Table 3** summarizes these common noncardiac causes.

Review of the Related Literature

Research about palpitations shows that they are a common reason for visits to the Emergency Department (ED)[5] and that the cause of the palpitations is varied from benign to life-threatening.[1,3] A study by Probst and colleagues[5] to determine the prevalence, demographic characteristics, and admission rates was conducted using the ED component of the National Hospital Ambulatory Medical Care Survey for 2001 through 2010, for patient visits whose chief complaint was palpitations. The researchers found that approximately 684,000 patients had a chief complaint of "palpitations," which represents a national prevalence of 5.8 per 1000 ED visits or 0.58%.

In a separate study, Weber and Kapoor[3] explored: "(a) the etiologies of palpitations, (b) the usefulness of diagnostic tests in determining the etiologies of palpitations, and (c) the outcomes of patients with palpitations" of patients who presented to a university medical center with the complaint of palpitations. A cohort of 196 patients was included in the study; each patient underwent a clinical interview and a psychiatric screening, and had their charts reviewed. The researchers were able to determine the cause of palpitations for 84% of the patients included in the study. More specifically, it was estimated that patients present with palpitations for the following reasons: (a) 43% were considered cardiac in nature, (b) 31% were related to a psychiatric cause, (c) 16% were due to unknown causes, and (d) 10% were due to miscellaneous causes.

Table 2 Cardiac causes of palpitations	
Ventricular	• Premature ventricular contractions • Ventricular tachycardia or fibrillation
High-output states	• Anemia • Arteriovenous fistula • Beriberi • Paget disease • Pregnancy
Structural abnormalities	• Acute left ventricular failure • Aortic aneurysm • Atrial myxoma • Cardiomegaly • Congenital heart disease
Miscellaneous	• Sinus tachycardia • Brugada syndrome • Postural orthostatic tachycardia syndrome (POTS)

Box 1
Brugada syndrome

- Genetic disease characterized by specific EKG changes and an increased risk of sudden cardiac death in male patients
- This syndrome has been recognized since 1992
- Patients can present with symptoms such as palpitations and syncope or be totally asymptomatic
- Characteristic EKG pattern is persistent ST elevations in leads V1-V3 with a right bundle branch block appearance with or without the terminal S waves in the lateral leads
- A prolongation of the PR interval is frequently seen
- An implantable cardioverter defibrillator is the only effective treatment to date

Data from Jellins J, Milanovic M, Taitz DJ, et al. Brugada syndrome. Hong Kong Med J 2013;19(2):159–67.

HISTORY AND PHYSICAL EXAMINATION FINDINGS

Obtaining a complete history is perhaps the most important step in determining the cause of palpitations. When diagnosing the cause of palpitations in a patient, it is helpful to know how they start and stop, that is, do they begin and end abruptly or not. It is also important to determine whether they are regular and the approximate rate during an episode.

History

The patient's description of the palpitations may be helpful in determining the cause. For example, palpitations associated with anxiety may be described by the patient as (a) a lump in the throat, (b) tingling in the hands and face, or (c) increased rate of breathing or hyperventilation. In comparison, palpitations that start and end abruptly usually indicate atrial or ventricular tachyarrhythmias.[7,8] Palpitations that have a more gradual onset usually indicate benign causes, such as sinus tachycardia during exercise or anxiety.[6]

Palpations associated with a pounding feeling in the neck may be caused by AV dissociation producing contractions of the atria against closed tricuspid and mitral valves,[7] producing cannon A waves that are perceived as neck pulsations.[6] The

---

Box 2
Postural orthostatic tachycardia syndrome

- Cardiac condition often associated with palpitations
- Type of orthostatic intolerance that is associated with the presence of tachycardia on standing
- Generally defined by a heart rate increase of 30 bpm or a rate that exceeds 120 bpm occurs within the first 10 minutes of standing
- Not associated with other chronic conditions such as prolonged bed rest or medications that diminish vascular tone

Data from Grubb B. Clinician update—postural tachycardia syndrome. Circulation 2008;117:2814–7.

Box 3
Cardiac conditions more commonly found in women

- Gender differences are noted in the cause and treatment of palpitations. The following conditions are more common in women:
  - Congenital long QT syndrome
  - Postural orthostatic tachycardia
- Nodal re-entry is the most common cause for paroxysmal supraventricular tachycardia in women.
- Women also have higher complication rates with invasive cardiac procedures and possible reduced benefit from implantable cardioverter defibrillator.

Data from Grubb B. Clinician update—postural tachycardia syndrome. Circulation 2008;117:2814–7.

---

sensation of rapid and regular pounding in the neck is most typical of re-entrant supraventricular arrhythmias, particularly AV nodal tachycardia.[6]

Palpitations associated with syncope can represent ventricular tachycardia, supraventricular tachycardia, or other cardiac arrhythmias. Palpitations associated angina may suggest myocardial ischemia precipitated by an increased oxygen demand, secondary to a rapid heart rate.[8]

Gathering information about the use of over-the-counter medications may also be crucial for trying to uncover a cause. Sympathomimetic agents found in allergy and cold medications as well as diet pills could all be a precipitating cause of palpitations.[7,9]

Physical Examination and Laboratory Tests

Certain findings on routine examination, if detected, may be helpful. General signs of anxiety such as tremors or nervous mannerisms; abnormal vital signs; pale skin; exophthalmos; goiter; jugular venous distention; carotid bruits; diminished carotid

---

Table 3
Noncardiac causes of palpitations

Metabolic	• Hyperthyroidism • Hypoglycemia • Hypocalcemia • Hyperkalemia • Hypokalemia • Hyperkalemia • Hypomagnesemia • Hypermagnesemia • Pheochromocytoma
Drug induced	• Alcohol • Amphetamines • Anticholinergic agents • Caffeine • Nicotine • Cocaine • Epinephrine
Psychiatric	• Generalized anxiety • Panic disorder • Somatization disorder

upstroke; heart murmurs; gallops and clicks; wheezes; rales; lower extremity edema; or calf tenderness can all be clues of the source of the palpitations.[4] Unfortunately, very often the patient who presents to the office does not currently have the symptoms of palpitations, and the physical examination does not offer many clues or insights into the underlying cause. Thus, often the diagnosis is not made through a routine examination or electrocardiogram (EKG).

Laboratory studies based on history and physical examination, such as hemoglobin and hematocrit, serum glucose levels, electrolyte levels, and thyroid function tests, may be relevant.[4] An EKG in the office is often nondiagnostic but it may show evidence of long QT syndrome, left ventricular hypertrophy, Q waves, short PR intervals or delta waves, and bundle branch blocks.[9]

ADDITIONAL TESTING FOR CARDIAC ARRHYTHMIAS

Even with a combination of history, physical examination, laboratory tests, and EKG, there are many times when the cause of the palpitations cannot be uncovered. However, if there is concern for a cardiac cause such as an arrhythmia, there are several outpatient ambulatory options that are available.

Holter Monitor

The Holter monitor is the method that is best used for palpitations that are found on a daily basis. A patient is asked to continue usual activities and record symptoms in a notebook. The 24-hour rhythm strip is analyzed to compare timing of symptoms and activity on the rhythm strip. If the patient has symptoms but there are no abnormalities on the rhythm strip, then a cardiac cause is less likely.[4]

Transtelephonic Electrocardiographic Monitoring

Also known as an event monitor or recorder, the transtelephonic electrocardiographic monitor is a handheld device applied to a patient's precordium. When symptoms occur, the patient presses a button to record about 30 seconds of cardiac rhythm. These rhythms are stored in a device and transmitted over the phone for printing and interpretation. Newer devices have memory loops that record rhythm data 2 minutes before the device is activated. These newer devices are more diagnostic and cost-effective then Holter monitors in patients with less frequent palpitations.[10]

Mobile Cardiac Outpatient Telemetry System

- If a patient has daily palpitations and is able to activate a monitor and transmit the data, then a short-term event monitor can be used. If the episodes are infrequent but last long enough to activate the monitor reliably, then a nonlooping event monitor can be used. If the episodes are infrequent and do not last long enough, then a continuous looping or real-time continuous device, such as a Mobile Cardiac Outpatient Telemetry system (MCOT), can be used.[11]
- The MCOT has 2 leads instead of 1 lead for monitoring. External loop recorders require patient activation, whereas MCOT does not. Information from MCOT goes straight to a central station. The external loop recorder requires the patient to transmit telephonically by the patient. MCOT patients receive a pocket-sized wireless recorder/personal digital assistant and installation of a home Internet base unit. Rhythm strips are recorded continuously and automatically transmitted wirelessly via an integrated cellular modem. EKGs are screened 24 hours a day by a central station with immediate referral to the physicians for evaluation of rate and rhythm changes in correlation with symptoms.[11]

Implantable Cardiac Monitors

The patient's EKG should be continuously monitored and real-time analysis performed for up to 36 months. The current clinical use of implantable cardiac monitors (ICMs) relate to the evaluation of transitory symptoms of difficult-to-explain palpitations or syncope. Inadequate patient compliance and patient discomfort and complexity have been an issue with the external recording devices. ICMs are smaller than a pacemaker, and once programmed, continuously monitor the patient's EKG and perform long-term and continuous analysis of the heart rhythm.[12]

Treadmill Exercise Testing

Treadmill exercise testing is helpful in patients with palpitations associated with exertion and risk factors for ischemic heart disease.[9]

Echocardiography

Echocardiography can be used to assess ventricular function and determine the presence or absence of valvular diseases. Echocardiography may be particularly helpful in young people or athletes with unexplained palpitations and could help establish the diagnosis of mitral valve prolapse or hypertrophic cardiomyopathy.[9]

Electrophysiologic Studies

Electrophysiologic studies (EPS) may be helpful for patients with a rapid pulse rate but normal EKG findings and for patients with palpitations preceding syncope. Patients with supraventricular tachycardia that is frequent and not controlled with medical treatment may benefit from radiofrequency ablation. If EPS reveals an inducible arrhythmia, ablation or placement of an implantable defibrillator can improve prognosis.[9]

Review of the Related Literature

In the aforementioned study by Weber and Kapoor,[3] researchers explored the usefulness of diagnostic tests in determining the causes of palpitations of patients who presented to a university medical center with the complaint of palpitations. The investigators found that patient history and physical examination data, along with the EKG or laboratory data, provided sufficient information to determine causes in 40% of the patients who participated in the study.

In comparison, a subsequent study by Hoefman and colleagues[10] explored the ability of general practitioners to determine the existence of a cardiac arrhythmia in patients who complained of palpitations and light-headedness. The researchers also investigated which signs and symptoms were used by physicians to predict the presence of arrhythmias as well as which were actually related to the existence of an arrhythmia. A cohort of 127 patients presenting to general practitioners in the Netherlands with symptoms of light-headedness and/or palpitations was included in this study. Patients underwent a physical examination, history, and EKG. The physicians' predication of the patient having an arrhythmia was compared with the results of a 30-day continuous event recording. The investigators found no correlation between the general practitioners' prediction of cardiac arrhythmia risk and the actual diagnosis of cardiac arrhythmia. The researchers concluded that general practitioners should have a low threshold for referring patients for additional cardiac testing when they present with symptoms of palpitations or light-headedness.

In another study by Hoefman and colleagues,[10] the researchers conducted a study that evaluated whether using event recorders affected these patients' anxiety and quality of life. The investigators noted that the continuous event recorder (CER) has proven to be successful in diagnosing causes of palpitations, but there was concern about the effects on quality of life. Therefore, they conducted a randomized controlled trial to assess this impact: one group carried the CER for 4 weeks, whereas the usual care group did not. The researchers found that the CER did not negatively influence anxiety or quality of life.

Hoefman and colleagues[11] explored the time needed for patient-activated CER to be a useful diagnostic tool in patients with palpitations or dizziness. They prospectively evaluated the time until diagnosis using CER in patients with symptoms of palpitations or dizziness in general practice. Patients ($N = 127$) received a CER up to 30 days. Of this group, 104 patients recorded events, and of this group, 78% ($n = 83$) demonstrated an arrhythmia. After 2 weeks, researchers were able to establish 75% of all diagnoses and 83.3% of all clinically relevant diagnoses. The investigators determined that a minimum recording time of 2 weeks seems necessary to determine most cardiac diagnoses.

Another study by Rothman and colleagues[12] compared the effectiveness of an MCOT to a patient-activated external loop for evaluating symptoms suspected to be due to an arrhythmia. Patients who reported symptoms of syncope, presyncope, or severe palpitations and had a nondiagnostic 24-hour Holter monitor were randomly assigned to the loop or MCOT group for up to 30 days. The researchers found that the MCOT (41%) provided a significantly higher yield than standard cardiac loop (15%) in patients with symptoms suggestive of a significant cardiac event.

A separate study by Locati and colleagues[13] looked at the use of extended external loop recorders for the diagnosis of unexplained syncope, presyncope, and sustained palpitations. The investigators found the diagnostic value of the external loop recorder in this group is similar to that of an implantable loop recorder using the same timeframe. They concluded that the external loop recorder could be considered before the use of the more invasive internal loop recorder.

DIAGNOSTIC DILEMMA: SUMMARY

Attempting to determine the underlying cause for a patient's complaint of palpitations is necessary in order to provide the appropriate therapy and/or reassurance. There is a wide range of reasons for palpitations that extend from benign to truly life-threatening conditions. It is crucial to obtain the proper history, physical examination, laboratory tests, and possible outpatient cardiac ambulatory tests to rule out some of these potentially life-threatening possibilities. If an arrhythmia is present, it should be taken seriously because it could be a sign of another organic, cardiac, or metabolic problem. Most patients can be clinically evaluated as an outpatient. There are times when admitting a patient for further evaluation is necessary, and these include palpitations associated with syncope, uncontrolled arrhythmias, hemodynamic compromise, and angina. In general, treating the cause of the palpitations can reduce or eliminate their occurrence. Palpitations are nonspecific symptoms that do not necessarily imply underlying serious heart disease but do raise concerns on the part of the patient and the physician.

The nonspecific case at the beginning of this article highlights the conundrum that primary care providers often face in the age of cost-conscious care. The physician really needs to perform a comprehensive history and understand the possible reasons for the initial complaint. Much of this may require an in-depth review of systems and understanding of a patient's concern. Like any other medical evaluation, the patient will need to understand the various possibilities and a certain amount of shared decision making will be required, especially since there are a wide variety of diagnostic tests that are available to a primary care physician. Even gender differences were found in regard to treatment responses and complication rates. It is also imperative that physicians have an understanding of all the outpatient devices that are available regarding the ability to detect arrhythmias because each has their own special nuances and cost associated with them. For most instances, the use of external devices is sufficient compared with internal devices. EPS studies are usually reserved for arrhythmias that are life threatening or recalcitrant to standard antiarrhythmic medications.

REFERENCES

1. Summerton M, Mann S, Rigby A, et al. New-onset palpitations in general practice: assessing the discriminant value of items within the clinical history. Fam Pract 2001;18(4):383–92.
2. Merriam Webster dictionary. Available at: http://www.merriam-webster.com/dictionary/palpitation. Accessed November 10, 2015.
3. Weber BE, Kapoor WN. Evaluation and outcomes of patients with palpitations. Am J Med 1996;100(2):138–48 [Erratum appears in Am J Med 1997;103(1):86].
4. Yalamanchili M, Khurana A, Smaha L. Evaluation of palpitations: etiology and diagnostic methods. Hospital Physician 2003;39(1):53–7.
5. Probst MA, Mower WR, Kanzaria HK, et al. Analysis of emergency department visits for palpitations (from the National Hospital Ambulatory Medical Care Survey). Am J Cardiol 2014;113(10):1685–90.
6. Ehlers A, Mayou R, Springings D, et al. Psychological and perceptual factors associated with arrhythmias and benign palpitations. Psychosom Med 2000;62: 693–702.
7. Archer TP, Schaal SF, Mazzaferri EL. Palpitations in a middle aged woman. Hosp Pract (1995) 1999;34:111–4, 118.
8. Pickett CC, Zimetbaum PJ. Palpitations: a proper evaluation and approach to effective medical therapy. Curr Cardiol Rep 2005;7:362–7.
9. Wexler RK, Pleister A, Raman S. Outpatient approach to palpitations. Am Fam Physician 2011;84(1):63–9.
10. Hoefman E, Boer KR, van Weert HC, et al. Predictive value of history taking and physical examination in diagnosing arrhythmias in general practice. Fam Pract 2007;24(6):636–41.
11. Hoefman E, van Weert HC, Boer KR, et al. Optimal duration of event recording for diagnosis of arrhythmias in patients with palpitations and light-headedness in the general practice. Fam Pract 2007;24(1):11–3.
12. Rothman SA, Laughlin JC, Seltzer J, et al. The diagnosis of cardiac arrhythmias: a prospective multi-center randomized study comparing mobile cardiac outpatient telemetry versus standard loop event monitoring. J Cardiovasc Electrophysiol 2007;18(3):241–7.
13. Locati ET, Vechhi AM, Vargiu S, et al. Role of extended external loop recorders for the diagnosis of unexplained syncope, pre-syncope, and sustained palpitations. Europace 2014;16(6):914–22.

Utility of Echocardiogram in the Evaluation of Heart Murmurs

Padmanabhan Premkumar, MD

KEYWORDS

- Murmur • Valvular heart disease • Echocardiogram • Primary care
- Cost-effective care

KEY POINTS

- Heart murmurs are a common occurrence in most patient populations in the United States.
- A complete cardiac physical examination remains the mainstay of initial assessment of heart murmurs.
- Careful consideration should be given regarding the ordering of an echocardiogram, relying on both evidence-based medicine and appropriate use criteria.

INTRODUCTION

Valvular heart disease (VHD) is a common cause of mortality and morbidity in the United States.[1,2] With an aging population, degenerative heart valves are a common clinical problem for primary care physicians. Many patients with VHD remain asymptomatic until the onset of underlying medical conditions that may precipitate the sequelae of their heart condition.[2] Varied clinical presentations from shortness of breath to syncope underlie some of the complications associated with this disease process. Early detection can lead to appropriate management decisions in potentially seriously ill patients.[2]

With its advent in the 1950s, echocardiography has become a fundamental part of cardiac evaluation and is the second most frequently performed diagnostic cardiac procedure.[3] The term echocardiography refers to the evaluation of the cardiac structures and function with the utility of ultrasound.[3] The ultra frequency sound waves along with Doppler have allowed for visual characterization of true cardiac abnormality. From its one-dimensional views to its evolution into 2-dimensional modality using either the thoracic or the transesophageal approach, it has significant capability in

The author does not have any financial disclosures.
Department of Medicine, Hartford Hospital, 85 Seymour Street, Hartford, CT 06102, USA
E-mail address: padmanabhan.premkumar@hhchealth.org

Med Clin N Am 100 (2016) 991–1001
http://dx.doi.org/10.1016/j.mcna.2016.04.005
medical.theclinics.com
0025-7125/16/$ – see front matter © 2016 Elsevier Inc. All rights reserved.

determining hemodynamics and flow.[4] In fact, ultrasound has evolved to become point of care in standard clinical practice conditions.

Echocardiography is a versatile imaging modality whose widespread use has fostered growing concern for its overuse and led to the development of appropriate use criteria (AUC).[5] National trends based on Medicare data show that use of echocardiograms (transthoracic [TTE] and transesophageal [TEE]) increased by 7.7% from 1999 to 2004, and it nearly doubled from 1999 to 2008.[1,5] Given the alarming trends in the cost of health care and the increasing frequency in the ordering of echocardiograms, judicious use of clinical guidelines and determinations based on signs and symptoms elicited during a thorough history and physical examination should guide the decision-making process in reference to these diagnostic procedures.

The cardiac physical examination still remains the mainstay in making the diagnosis of VHD and potential referral for an echocardiogram. The diagnosis of a murmur begins with the careful assessment of its characteristics and response to bedside maneuvers.[6] The prevalence of heart murmurs varies among different populations with benign or functional murmurs being quite common.[7] The most frequent murmur in the population is a systolic murmur, which occurs in 80% to 96% of children and 15% to 44% of adults.[8] Among elderly outpatients, the prevalence of systolic murmurs ranges from almost 29% to 60%, and results of echocardiography are normal in 44% to 100% of cases.[7] The asymptomatic nature of this prevalent condition emphasizes the need for continued focus on the physical examination, which then allows for guidelines to help dictate standard of care.

PHYSICAL EXAMINATION

Heart murmurs are typically caused by audible vibrations due to turbulent blood flow across the valve and can indicate an underlying abnormality.[9] Murmurs are based on their timing in the cardiac cycle. Systolic murmurs begin with or after the first heart sound (S_1) and terminate at or before the component of the second heart sound (S_2) that corresponds to the site of origin (left or right, respectively).[10,11] Diastolic murmurs begin with or after the associated component of S_2 and end at or before the subsequent S_1. The duration of a heart murmur is reflected by the pressure difference across the chambers or vessels that in turn dictate flow, turbulence, and intensity of the murmur.[10,11] The configuration of a heart murmur involves the pressure difference across the various cycles between the involved chambers of the heart.[10,11] Finally, the intensity of the heart murmur is graded from scale of I through VI, ranging from very soft to a murmur being loud enough to be heard even with the stethoscope not in contact with the chest.[11] Murmur evaluation also includes dynamic auscultation (bedside maneuvers)[7] and several nonauscultatory components, such as[7]

- Blood pressure (including pulse pressure), pulse, respiration
- Carotid pulse, jugular veins
- Precordial palpation
- Additional heart sounds (including clicks, ejection sounds, and splitting of S_2, S_3, S_4)
- Abdominal examination (ascites)
- Extremities (edema)

Murmurs are generally classified as either functional (benign in nature, without underlying abnormality) or organic.[7] Although many murmurs are functional in origin, there may be tremendous variability in distinguishing it from true organic abnormality.

Characteristics of benign/functional murmurs as defined by the American College of Cardiology (ACC)/American Heart Association (AHA)[6] guidelines are as follows:
Presence of

- Systolic murmur of short duration
- Grade 1 or 2 in intensity at the left sternal border
- Systolic ejection pattern
- A normal S2

Absence of

- Abnormal sounds or murmurs
- Left ventricular hypertrophy or dilatation
- Thrills
- Increase in intensity with the Valsalva maneuver

Murmurs with these features along with normal electrocardiogram tracing and plain chest radiographs are infrequently associated with cardiac abnormality.[6]

The evidence regarding continued use of the cardiac physical examination as the mainstay in the evaluation of VHD is abundant. Despite the growing trend in the utilization of ultrasound at point of care, it should not replace the physical examination in the initial diagnostic assessment. Best efforts in order to achieve high value, cost-conscious care in the assessment of patients with heart murmurs should focus on the continued teaching, practice, and mastery of the cardiac examination. In fact, the guidelines and criteria that guide referrals for echocardiograms require pertinent details from the physical examination. Several studies have compared the utility of the cardiac physical examination to echocardiograms in the evaluation of VHD.

Shry and colleagues[12] conducted a study enrolling 72 military patients who were referred to the cardiology clinic with an abnormal precordial examination. Those with previously known abnormal echocardiograms or being referred for other cardiac complaints were excluded from the study. The utility of ACC/AHA guidelines was evaluated in murmur detection in a relatively young, healthy population. The results of the study showed that the cardiac examination had an almost 100% negative predictive value for cardiac valvular abnormality on echocardiography in patients with normal cardiac examinations. Approximately 30 patients did not meet ACC/AHA guidelines for an innocent murmur, yet even in this population, only 30% had an abnormal echocardiogram. The investigators concluded that a stepped approach following ACC/AHA guidelines toward echocardiography would have prevented almost 58% of the echocardiograms in this study.[12]

Roldan and colleagues[13] prospectively studied 143 subjects to determine the accuracy of cardiovascular physical examination in diagnosing asymptomatic VHD. Approximately 75 patients in the study had disease known to produce VHD, whereas 68 patients were described as normal. Cardiac physical examination was compared with TEE in detecting clinically significant heart murmurs. The results of the study concluded that the TEE detected 33 patients (23%) with at least one form of VHD, while physical examination detected 25 patients (17%) in this study population. Overall, the dynamic cardiac examination had a sensitivity of 70% and specificity of 98% in this study. Only 2 of the 8 patients in the TEE group that were identified with VHD outside the physical examination cohort actually had clinically significant VHD. The overall conclusion of the study was that the physical examination still remains the gold standard in assessing cardiac murmurs rather than routine application of echocardiography.[13]

Attenhofer Jost and colleagues[8] conducted a similar study, involving 100 patients, to determine whether physical examination can reliably assess systolic murmurs of various causes. The diagnostic accuracy of the physical examination was validated using echocardiography in all 100 patients. Nearly 21% of the patients had completely normal echocardiographic findings. The sensitivity of the physical examination approached almost 79% in detecting significant heart disease, and a functional murmur could be recognized with a sensitivity of 67%. There was some discrepancy in the physical examination and echocardiogram in patients with severe aortic stenosis, low-flow states, and those patients with multiple murmurs. Overall, the study concluded that physical examinations could routinely differentiate between functional and organic murmurs. They also determined that although physical examination remains the first-line assessment, echocardiograms offer an additional diagnostic tool in situations of clinical uncertainty.[8]

Summary of the studies mentioned above are shown in **Table 1**.

Table 1 Summary of studies showing importance of physical examination in assessing valvular heart disease			
Study	Purpose	Number of Patients (N)	Results
Shry et al,[12] 2001	Utility of ACC/AHA guidelines in screening patients with possible valvular abnormality[8]	72	Conclusion: published guidelines were useful in defining abnormal pathology and obviating additional testing
Roldan et al,[13] 1996	Utility of "dynamic cardiac examination" in detecting VHD[9]	143	Conclusion: cardiac physical examination had tremendous clinical utility and was recommended as the first test of choice in routine application
Attenhofer Jost et al,[8] 2000	Utility of physical examination compared with echocardiograms in detecting the cause of systolic murmurs[6]	100	• Physical examinations were useful in characterizing the difference between functional and organic murmurs • Conclusion: with only 2% of the VHDs being missed, cardiac physical examinations were just as valuable as modern imaging in detecting abnormality

ECHOCARDIOGRAPHY AND CLINICAL GUIDELINES

TTE has become the gold standard in the evaluation of clinically significant VHD.[6] Its relatively low cost, absence of radiation, and portability has allowed it to have significant utility in all facets of medicine.[5] Unfortunately, its accessibility and ease of use have also created overuse[5] and the need to create standardized guidelines. Currently, the ACC/AHA guidelines[6] along with AUC allow for objective ordering of TTE/TEE based on clinical symptoms and findings. In response to the dramatic increase in imaging studies over the past decade, the ACC in conjunction with American Society of Echocardiography and other imaging subspecialty societies developed the AUC for TTE.[14] Initially developed in 2007 and updated in 2011, the AUC provides specific criteria for rational use of imaging studies that impact physician decision-making.[14]

The ACC/AHA Guidelines for echocardiogram evaluation of heart murmurs include the following:

- Define the primary lesion and its cause and judge its severity
- Define hemodynamics
- Detect coexisting abnormalities
- Detect lesions secondary to the primary lesion
- Evaluate cardiac size and function
- Establish a reference for future observations
- Re-evaluate a patient after an intervention

The major indications based on the available guidelines are listed in **Table 2**. The guidelines are adopted from the ACC/AHA[6] along with the AUC[15] for the use of TTEs in the evaluation of VHD.

Table 2
Comparison of American College of Cardiology/American Heart Association Guidelines with appropriate use criteria regarding indications for echocardiogram use

ACC/AHA Guidelines[6]	Appropriate Use Criteria[15]
Murmur in a patient with cardiorespiratory symptoms (class I)	Initial evaluation when there is a reasonable suspicion of valvular or structural heart disease
Murmur in an asymptomatic patient if the clinical features indicate at least a moderate probability that the murmur is reflective of structural heart disease (class I)	Re-evaluation of known VHD with a change in clinical status or cardiac examination or to guide therapy
Murmur in an asymptomatic patient in whom there is a low probability of heart disease but in whom the diagnosis of heart disease cannot be reasonably excluded by the standard cardiovascular clinical evaluation (class IIa)	

Class I: conditions for which there is evidence and/or general agreement that a given procedure or treatment is useful and effective; class II: conditions for which there is conflicting evidence and/or a divergence of opinion about the usefulness/efficacy of a procedure or treatment; class IIa: weight of evidence/opinion is in favor of usefulness/efficacy.

Echocardiography has the distinct advantage of defining the underlying abnormality of murmurs when they are not considered to be function or benign; however, its utility with untrained noncardiologists is an important question to answer. Several studies have looked at ultrasound use in the hands of inexperienced personnel and compared them to routine bedside cardiovascular examinations. In fact, Kobal and colleagues[16] conducted a study in 2005 comparing the effectiveness of hand-carried ultrasound with bedside physical examinations. Third-year medical students received 18 hours of training for 3 weeks, of which 14 hours were spent obtaining practical experience using the hand-held device The study included 61 patients comparing cardiovascular diagnoses by medical students using handheld ultrasound with standard physical examinations by trained cardiologists. All patients underwent echocardiography to determine the existence of any cardiac abnormality. Of the 239 abnormal findings identified by standard echocardiography, students recognized 75% and cardiologists identified 49%. Subset analysis of the cardiac abnormalities in the study included VHD. The students using the handheld technology in the study had a sensitivity of 89% compared with cardiologists (50%) for the diagnosis of organic valvular lesions (P value <.001). The results of the study indicated that brief bedside ultrasound training was superior to cardiac physical examinations in detection of valvular disease.[16]

Another study in 2003 conducted by DeCara and colleagues[17] looked at the use of ultrasound devices by internal medicine residents without formal training in echocardiography. They compared 300 patients who received formal echocardiograms with bedside ultrasonography by these residents. Although resident and echocardiographer-performed scans had similar sensitivity and specificity, the positive predictive value was much higher for the echocardiographer-performed scans. Clinically important findings showed slightly, but significantly, higher sensitivity for echocardiographer-performed scans. They concluded that training guidelines and competency evaluation are needed if these devices are to be used for clinical decision making.[17]

Ultrasound has graduated to become standard of care in several critical areas requiring immediate decision making. Guidelines now exist for point-of-care ultrasound for critically ill patients. The degree of detail in these situations allows for even a less experienced hand to make logical medical decisions. However, decisions regarding degree of valvular stenosis or regurgitation that impact diagnosis and treatment likely require more experience and training.

COMMON HEART MURMURS
Native Valve Stenosis

Aortic stenosis
Common causes include bicuspid aortic valve with degenerative calcification, deterioration of trileaflet valve, and rheumatic heart disease.[2,4,9]

Clinical manifestations of aortic stenosis include exertional dyspnea, left ventricular dysfunction, angina, and syncope. Diagnostic features on physical exam and echocardiography indications for Aortic stenosis are listed in **Table 3**.[2,4,9]

Table 3
Aortic stenosis with diagnostic features on physical examination and echocardiogram along with indications based on American College of Cardiology/American Heart Association Guidelines

Murmur	Physical Examination[2,4,9]	Echocardiographic Findings[2,4,9]	ACC/AHA Guidelines[6]
Aortic stenosis	• Weak/delayed arterial pulses with carotid thrill • Double apical impulse • A₂ soft or absent • S4 common Typically crescendo decrescendo murmur with systolic thrill loudest at the right second intercostal space with radiation to the carotids and sometimes apex	• Left ventricular hypertrophy • Thickening of AV cusps with reduced opening Doppler indicates transvalvular gradients and aortic valve areas	Diagnosis; assessment of hemodynamic severity Assessment of left ventricular and right ventricular size/function, and/or hemodynamics

Mitral stenosis
Common causes include rheumatic heart disease and congenital mitral stenosis (MS; rare—mainly in children).

Clinical manifestations include dyspnea, pulmonary edema precipitated by respiratory infection, atrial fibrillation, or other conditions causing tachycardia Diagnostic features on physical exam and echocardiography indications for Mitral stenosis are listed in **Table 4**.[2,4,9]

Table 4
Mitral stenosis with diagnostic features on physical examination and echocardiogram along with indications based on American College of Cardiology/American Heart Association Guidelines

Murmur	Physical Examination[2,4,9]	Echocardiographic Findings[2,4,9]	ACC/AHA Guidelines[6]
Mitral stenosis	• Opening snap follows A_2 • Palpable S1 • Right ventricular heave Typically low-pitched diastolic rumbling heard loudest at the apex In severe MS, murmur throughout diastole with presystolic accentuation in sinus rhythm	• Characteristic inadequate separation with calcification and thickening of the leaflets • Left atrial enlargement Doppler indicates transvalvular gradient, mitral valve area, and degree of pulmonary hypertension	Diagnosis; assessment of hemodynamic severity Assessment of left ventricular and right ventricular size/ function and/or hemodynamics

Prognostic information from hemodynamic response to exercise and/or morphologic characteristics from the echocardiogram helps drive selection of treatment options and further follow-up.[6] The AUC in 2011 has provided baseline options for follow-up in native valve stenosis:

Routine surveillance ($\geq$3 years) of mild valvular stenosis without a change in clinical status or cardiac examination[15]

Routine surveillance ($\geq$1 year) of moderate or severe valvular stenosis without a change in clinical status or cardiac examination[15]

Native Valve Regurgitation

Aortic regurgitation
Common causes include

Rheumatic heart disease
Bicuspid aortic valve
Endocarditis
Dilated aortic roots (aortic dissection/ankylosing spondylitis/syphilis)[9]

Clinical manifestations of aortic regurgitation include exertional dyspnea, angina pectoris, and pulmonary edema. In addition, water hammer pulse, wide pulse

Table 5
Aortic regurgitation with diagnostic features on physical examination and echocardiogram along with indications based on American College of Cardiology/American Heart Association Guidelines

Murmur	Physical Examination[2,4,9]	Echocardiographic Findings[2,4,9]	ACC/AHA Guidelines[6]
Aortic regurgitation	• A_2 soft or absent • S_3 present Diastolic blowing decrescendo murmur loudest along the left sternal border; possible systolic murmur with augmented blood flow	• Left atrial and left ventricular enlargement • Failure of aortic leaflets • Diastolic fluttering of mitral valve (high frequency) Doppler to quantify regurgitation	Diagnosis; assessment of hemodynamic severity Assessment of left ventricular and right ventricular size/ function, and/or hemodynamics

pressure, and capillary pulsation are characteristic features Diagnostic features on physical exam and echocardiography indications for Aortic regurgitation are listed in **Table 5.**[9]

Mitral regurgitation
Common causes include

Rheumatic heart disease
Papillary muscle dysfunction with coronary artery disease
Left ventricular dilatation
Mitral annular calcification, hypertrophic cardiomyopathy/endocarditis[9]

Clinical manifestations include fatigue, weakness, and exertional dyspnea Diagnostic features on physical exam and echocardiography indications for Mitral regurgitation are listed in **Table 6**.

Table 6
Mitral regurgitation with diagnostic features on physical examination and echocardiogram along with indications based on American College of Cardiology/American Heart Association Guidelines

Murmur	Physical Examination[2,4,9]	Echocardiographic Findings[2,4,9]	ACC/AHA Guidelines[6]
Mitral regurgitation	• S_1 diminished • Wide splitting of S_2 • S_3 heard • Brisk arterial upstroke Loud holosystolic murmur with mid diastolic rumble	• Large left atrium • Hyperdynamic left ventricle Doppler to assess severity of regurgitation and degree of pulmonary hypertension	Diagnosis; assessment of hemodynamic severity Assessment of left ventricular and right ventricular size/ function and/or hemodynamics

The best evidence for surveillance based on the AUC data shows that routine imaging (≥ 1 year) is indicated for moderate-to-severe valvular regurgitation without a change in clinical status or cardiac examination.[15]

TRANSESOPHAGEAL ECHOCARDIOGRAPHY

The TEE is an additional and more accurate test compared with the TTE given the proximity of the esophagus to the heart and the great vessels.[18] There are specific indications for the TEE primarily involving the evaluation of VHD. The clinical application of TEE includes the evaluation of native valve disease and prosthetic valve dysfunction. The guidelines for performing a comprehensive TEE based on the American Society of Echocardiography and Society of Anesthesiologists are as follows[18]:

- Evaluation of valvular structure and function to assess suitability for, and assist in planning of, an intervention
- To diagnose infective endocarditis with a moderate or high pretest probability (eg, staphylococcus bacteremia, fungemia, prosthetic heart valve, or intracardiac device)
- Re-evaluation of prior TEE finding for interval change (eg, resolution of vegetation after completion of antibiotic therapy) when a change in therapy is anticipated

COST TRENDS IN THE USE OF ECHOCARDIOGRAPHY

The use of echocardiograms has doubled during the past decade.[14] In fact, echocardiography constitutes half of all cardiac imaging services among Medicare beneficiaries in the United States.[14] In 2007, Pearlman and colleagues[19] conducted a study on evolving trends in echocardiography among Medicare beneficiaries, results of which indicated an annual growth rate of 7.7% in the use of echocardiograms. Although cardiology provided a large portion of the echocardiography services, most studies were ordered by primary care physicians and noncardiologists.[19] A review of Medicare services provided by cardiologists from 1999 to 2008 revealed that most of the growth in services was driven by the increase in noninvasive imaging.[1] In 2010, echocardiography contributed to 11% of the $1.1 billion in Medicare expenditures on imaging.[14] Per the "Choosing Wisely" campaign, a standard echocardiogram can cost $1000 to $2000, whereas a TEE can be $2000 or more.[20–23] The cost to the patient can include a copay of 10% to 50% even for those with insurance. Given the significant increase in utilization of echocardiography, the cost of the procedure both to the patient and to the overall health care expenditures, and the specific indications of when these studies should be used in the assessment of cardiac murmurs, judicious use of echocardiography referrals based on appropriate guidelines is highly recommended.

FUTURE CONSIDERATIONS/SUMMARY

The advancing age and overall longevity of the population increase the likelihood of degenerative valvular disease. When complications arise, the need for early detection and treatment is paramount to prevent significant morbidity. However, given the high rates of benign/functional murmurs, the need for clinicians to distinguish between these murmurs and those associated with clinical disease is necessary. Initial assessment of the heart murmurs should involve a thorough cardiac physical examination with appropriate maneuvers. Based on accurate characterization and response to these maneuvers, an echocardiogram may or may not be necessary. It is recommended that the appropriate society-based guidelines, as outlined, be followed to ensure cost-effective utilization of echocardiograms.

REFERENCES

1. Andrus BW, Welch HG. Medicare services provided by cardiologists in the United States: 1999-2008. Circ Cardiovasc Qual Outcomes 2012;5(1):31–6.
2. Sorrentino MJ. Valvular heart disease. Chapter 29. In: Hall JB, Schmidt GA, Wood LH, editors. Principles of critical care. 3rd edition. New York: McGraw-Hill; 2005. Available at: http://accessmedicine.mhmedical.com/content.aspx?bookid=361&Sectionid=39866396. Accessed November 26, 2015.
3. Palmeri ST, Cohen L, Shindler DM. Echocardiography. Chapter 1. In: Pahlm O, Wagner GS, editors. Multimodal cardiovascular imaging: principles and clinical applications. New York: McGraw-Hill; 2011. Available at: http://accessmedicine.mhmedical.com/content.aspx?bookid=382&Sectionid=40663652. Accessed November 26, 2015.
4. DeMaria AN, Blanchard DG. Echocardiography. Chapter 18. In: Fuster V, Walsh RA, Harrington RA, editors. Hurst's the heart. 13th edition. New York: McGraw-Hill; 2011. Available at: http://accessmedicine.mhmedical.com/content.aspx?bookid=376&Sectionid=40279744. Accessed November 28, 2015.
5. Papolos A, Narula J, Bavishi C, et al. U.S. hospital use of echocardiography. J Am Coll Cardiol 2016;67:502–11.

6. Cheitlin MD, Alpert JS, Armstrong WF, et al. ACC/AHA guidelines for the clinical application of echocardiography: executive summary. A report of the American College of Cardiology/American Heart Association Task Force on Practice Guidelines (Committee on Clinical Application of Echocardiography). Developed in collaboration with the American Society of Echocardiography. J Am Coll Cardiol 1997;29:862–79.

7. Shub C. Echocardiography or auscultation? How to evaluate systolic murmurs. Can Fam Physician 2003;49:163–7.

8. Attenhofer Jost CH, Turina J, Mayer K, et al. Echocardiography in the evaluation of systolic murmurs of unknown cause. Am J Med 2000;108:614–20.

9. Longo DL, Fauci AS, Kasper DL, et al. Valvular heart disease. In: Longo DL, Fauci AS, Kasper DL, et al, editors. Harrison's manual of medicine. 18th edition. New York: McGraw-Hill; 2013. Available at: http://accessmedicine.mhmedical.com/content.aspx?bookid=1140&Sectionid=63501912. Accessed November 26, 2015.

10. O'Gara PT, Loscalzo J. Approach to the patient with a heart murmur. In: Kasper D, Fauci A, Hauser S, et al, editors. Harrison's principles of internal medicine. 19th edition. New York: McGraw-Hill; 2015. Available at: http://accessmedicine.mhmedical.com/content.aspx?bookid=1130&Sectionid=66487549. Accessed February 25, 2016.

11. Walsh RA, O'Rourke RA, Shaver JA. The history, physical examination, and cardiac auscultation. Chapter 14. In: Fuster V, Walsh RA, Harrington RA, editors. Hurst's the heart. 13th edition. New York: McGraw-Hill; 2011. Available at: http://accessmedicine.mhmedical.com/content.aspx?bookid=376&Sectionid=40279740. Accessed February 25, 2016.

12. Shry EA, Smithers MA, Mascette AM. Auscultation versus echocardiography in a healthy population with precordial murmur. Am J Cardiol 2001;87:1428–30.

13. Roldan CA, Shively BK, Crawford MH. Value of the cardiovascular physical examination for detecting valvular heart disease in asymptomatic subjects. Am J Cardiol 1996;77:1327–31.

14. Matulevicius SA, Rohatgi A, Das SR, et al. Appropriate use and clinical impact of transthoracic echocardiography. JAMA Intern Med 2013;173(17):1600–7.

15. American College of Cardiology Foundation Appropriate Use Criteria Task Force, American Society of Echocardiography, American Heart Association, American Society of Nuclear Cardiology, Heart Failure Society of America; Heart Rhythm Society, Society for Cardiovascular Angiography and Interventions, Society of Critical Care Medicine, Society of Cardiovascular Computed Tomography, Society for Cardiovascular Magnetic Resonance, American College of Chest Physicians, Douglas PS, Garcia MJ, Haines DE, et al. ACCF/ASE/AHA/ASNC/HFSA/HRS/SCAI/SCCM/SCCT/SCMR 2011 Appropriate Use Criteria for Echocardiography: a report of the American College of Cardiology Foundation Appropriate Use Criteria Task Force, American Society of Echocardiography, American Heart Association, American Society of Nuclear Cardiology, Heart Failure Society of America, Heart Rhythm Society, Society for Cardiovascular Angiography and Interventions, Society of Critical Care Medicine, Society of Cardiovascular Computed Tomography, Society for Cardiovascular Magnetic Resonance American College of Chest Physicians. J Am Soc Echocardiogr 2011;24(3):229–67.

16. Kobal SL, Trento L, Baharami S, et al. Comparison of effectiveness of hand held ultrasound to bedside cardiovascular physical examination. Am J Cardiol 2005;96(7):1002–6.

17. DeCara JM, Lang RM, Koch R, et al. The use of small personal ultrasound devices by internists without formal training in echocardiography. Eur J Echocardiogr 2003;4(2):141–7.

18. Hahn RT, Abraham T, Adams MS, et al. Guidelines for performing a comprehensive transesophageal echocardiographic examination: recommendations from the American Society of Echocardiography and the Society of Cardiovascular Anesthesiologists. J Am Soc Echocardiogr 2013;26:921–64.

19. Pearlman AS, Ryan T, Picard MH, et al. Evolving trends in the use of echocardiography: a study of Medicare beneficiaries. J Am Coll Cardiol 2007;49(23): 2283–91.

20. Echocardiograms for heart valve disease. Choosing wisely website. 2012. Available at: http://www.choosingwisely.org/patient-resources/echocardiograms-for-heart-valve-disease/. Accessed February 23, 2016.

21. A data book: health care spending and the Medicare program. 2012. Available at: www.medpac.gov/documents/Jun12DataBookEntireReport.pdf. Accessed November 20, 2012.

22. Welch HG, Hayes KJ, Frost C. Repeat testing among Medicare beneficiaries. Arch Intern Med 2012;172(22):1745–51.

23. Douglas PS, Khandheria B, Stainback RF, et al, American College of Cardiology Foundation Quality Strategic Directions Committee Appropriateness Criteria Working Group, American Society of Echocardiography, American College of Emergency Physicians, American Society of Nuclear Cardiology, Society for Cardiovascular Angiography and Interventions, Society of Cardiovascular Computed Tomography, Society for Cardiovascular Magnetic Resonance, American College of Chest Physicians, Society of Critical Care Medicine. ACCF/ASE/ACEP/ASNC/ SCAI/SCCT/SCMR 2007 appropriateness criteria for transthoracic and transesophageal echocardiography: a report of the American College of Cardiology Foundation Quality Strategic Directions Committee Appropriateness Criteria Working Group, American Society of Echocardiography, American College of Emergency Physicians, American Society of Nuclear Cardiology, Society for Cardiovascular Angiography and Interventions, Society of Cardiovascular Computed Tomography, and the Society for Cardiovascular Magnetic Resonance endorsed by the American College of Chest Physicians and the Society of Critical Care Medicine. J Am Coll Cardiol 2007;50(2):187–204.

Avoiding Unnecessary Preoperative Testing

Matthew H. Rusk, MD

KEYWORDS

- Preoperative testing • Preoperative ECGs • Cataract surgery

KEY POINTS

- Preoperative laboratory testing is not indicated before cataract surgery.
- Routine urinalysis is not needed before surgery.
- Routine electrocardiograms are indicated preoperatively in selected patients only.
- Routine coagulation studies are not necessary before surgery.

INTRODUCTION

In general, preoperative testing is ordered with the hope of identifying potential unforeseen issues that may lead to complications from surgery. Enormous medical resources are used in the pursuit of this goal, yet there is little evidence indicating that such routine testing is of any real usefulness. All medical testing has an inherent rate of false positives that can lead to many difficulties for the testing physician and, more importantly, for patients. When tests are applied to an asymptomatic population, the rate of false-positive tests automatically goes up, which may lead to further testing. Many physicians inherently understand this but think that foregoing testing will expose them to medicolegal risks. Interestingly, many of these abnormal preoperative tests are not even followed up,[1] which paradoxically may expose the physician to more legal risk than if the studies had never been ordered in the first place. This article examines the utility of preoperative laboratory testing before cataract surgery, as well as the utility of the routine preoperative urinalysis, electrocardiogram (ECG), and coagulation studies.

PREOPERATIVE TESTING BEFORE CATARACT SURGERY

The risks involved in any operation depend on both the risk of the procedure and the patient's overall health. If the patient's health is excellent, the risk depends largely on

Disclosure Statement: The author has nothing to disclose.
Division of General Internal Medicine, Perelman School of Medicine at the University of Pennsylvania, 51 North 39th Street, Medical Arts Building, Suite 102, Philadelphia, PA 19104, USA
E-mail address: matthew.rusk@uphs.upenn.edu

Med Clin N Am 100 (2016) 1003–1008
http://dx.doi.org/10.1016/j.mcna.2016.04.011
0025-7125/16/$ – see front matter © 2016 Elsevier Inc. All rights reserved.

the nature of the procedure. If the procedural risk is extremely low, then the patient's overall health does not have much bearing on the outcome. Such is the case with cataract surgery. This surgery does not require general anesthesia and does not typically cause blood loss or hemodynamic challenges. Complications are generally limited to the eye itself. Nonetheless, cost estimates in the United States for preoperative testing before 2000 have suggested more than 150 million dollars yearly was spent on this dubious endeavor.[2]

Cataract surgery is the most commonly performed elective operation for Medicare beneficiaries in the United States[3] and, as a consequence, it generates a large number of preoperative consultations ordered by ophthalmologists. The procedure typically takes about 20 minutes and the risk of cardiac complications is less than 1%.[3] Solid evidence suggests that routine laboratory testing does not affect patient outcomes. As a result, such testing may not be justified and could be considered a misuse of medical resources.

The most convincing study analyzing the outcomes of preoperative testing before cataract surgery demonstrated no benefit to doing a standard battery of tests that included ECG and basic laboratory analysis (eg, complete blood count and serum electrolytes).[4] This trial randomized 18,189 subjects at 9 centers to a testing or nontesting strategy using an intention-to-treat analysis. Operative complications were measured and included both serious and nonserious events. Serious events included myocardial infarction or ischemia, congestive heart failure, hypertension or hypotension, arrhythmia, stroke or transient ischemic attack, respiratory failure or desaturation, or blood sugar excursions, including diabetic ketoacidosis or nonketotic hyperosmolar syndrome. Operative complications were assessed using a standardized form filled out by the anesthesiologist or nurse anesthetist. In addition, a study coordinator, using a standardized telephone interview, contacted the subject or the subject's family 1 week postoperative to ask about further postoperative complications.

The results revealed that cataract surgery was a very low-risk procedure in both groups of subjects, whether or not they underwent preoperative testing. Both groups had the same total event rate of 31.3 events per 1000 operations, with no intraoperative deaths reported. The rate of hospitalization per 1000 operations was 0.3 per 1000 operations in the tested group and 0.5 per 1000 operations in the nontested group. This small difference, however, was not statistically significant. The most commonly reported complications were hypertension and arrhythmia (mainly bradycardia), which accounted for 68% of the events in the testing group and 61% in the nontesting group. It should also be noted that these subjects were older (mean age of just under 75 years in both groups), with a fairly representative list of medical problems that would be expected in this age group.

In summary, this well-designed, large trial showed no benefit to preoperative testing for cataract surgery. Because cataract surgery is such a common operation, the cessation of routine testing would result in substantial cost savings without an increase in complications.

ROUTINE URINALYSIS IN THE PREOPERATIVE PERIOD

Routine urinalyses are commonly ordered before surgery in the hope that identifying asymptomatic urinary tract infections or urinary colonization, and treating them, will reduce the rate of perioperative infection. Nowhere is this more true than in orthopedics, and it is this setting for which the most data are available. Prosthetic joint infections can be a devastating complication of joint replacement surgery and it seems logical that treating asymptomatic urinary tract infections might lower the rate of bacteremia and subsequent seeding of the prosthetic joint. As logical as it seems, the available studies to date have shown no benefit to a screen and treat strategy before orthopedic surgery.

The largest study in this regard prospectively evaluated nearly 2500 subjects undergoing elective hip or knee replacement surgery in 3 different sites in Europe.[5] All subjects had a routine urine culture sent before surgery. The prevalence of asymptomatic bacteriuria was 12.1%, with a 2 to 1 predominance in women. Subjects were then assigned to antimicrobial therapy at the discretion of their physician in a nonrandomized fashion. Although the rate of joint infection in those with asymptomatic bacteriuria was higher than in those with sterile urine cultures (4.3% vs 1.4%, odds ratio 3.23, 95% confidence interval 1.67–6.27, $P = .001$), those who had treatment of their bacteriuria did not have fewer joint infections than those who did not have treatment. It is very important to point out that the pathogens isolated from prosthetic joint infections did not match any of those from the urine in those subjects who had antecedent asymptomatic bacteria. Although the trial was limited by the nonrandomization of antimicrobial therapy in those subjects with asymptomatic bacteriuria, the lack of correspondence between the urine isolate and the pathogen isolated from the prosthetic joint infection suggests there is no direct link. The investigators surmised that asymptomatic bacteriuria is more likely a marker of risk for infection than a direct cause of infection. Currently no consensus panels recommend routine urine cultures before surgery.

PREOPERATIVE ELECTROCARDIOGRAMS IN PATIENTS UNDERGOING SURGERY

There are no randomized controlled trials demonstrating that the use of ECGs as preoperative tests reduces operative complications or mortality. Nonetheless, there is evidence that an abnormal ECG predicts an increased rate of serious cardiac events. Expert consensus suggests that the ECG is useful in certain categories of patients or in those undergoing high-risk surgical procedures.

In a prospective observational cohort study of 345 subjects undergoing major surgery, an abnormal ECG was found in roughly 40% of those studied.[6] In this relatively small, nonrandomized trial, a major adverse cardiac event (MACE) was defined as a nonfatal myocardial infarction or death related to cardiac causes. The study noted a relatively high event rate of 13.3%. The rate of MACE in subjects with an abnormal ECG was 21.6% versus 8.3% in those with a normal ECG. In particular, left ventricular strain and a prolonged QTc were predictive of an adverse event.

Other ECG changes also predict adverse events in patients with known coronary artery disease undergoing major noncardiac surgery. In a prospective cohort study of 172 subjects having such surgery, preoperative ST segment changes and an elevated heart rate were both found to be independent risk factors for mortality.[7]

Although the preoperative ECG may have predictive power with respect to outcomes, there is no randomized controlled trial showing that the use of ECG led to a reduction in the overall event rate even if it is predictive of a higher risk. It is this predictive power, however, that gets the preoperative ECG a positive recommendation in various guidelines for certain patients. The most widely accepted guidelines come from the 2014 American College of Cardiology/American Heart Association (ACC/AHA).[8] These give clear recommendations for the selected use of preoperative ECGs. The guidelines use a rating system in which interventions are categorized as class I, class IIa, class IIb, or class III. Class I interventions should be performed, class IIb interventions are reasonable to be performed, and class IIb interventions may be considered. Class III interventions are not recommended and have either no benefit or may actually cause harm. The guidelines rate the quality of evidence for these recommendations as either A, B, or C. Interventions with an A rating have the highest quality evidence and are generally based on the results of multiple randomized trials in different populations. Level B ratings are in limited populations and the data are derived from a single randomized controlled trial or nonrandomized trials. Level C evidence comes from very limited populations with only consensus opinion or case studies backing that recommendation.

According to these guidelines, preoperative ECGs are not recommended for procedures that are considered low-risk. This recommendation stands even if the patient has antecedent cardiac disease or cardiac risk factors that would put him or her at higher risk. The guidelines give the intervention a class III rating, which means no benefit based on evidence that is rated as B in quality.

The guidelines do, however, recommend preoperative ECGs in patients undergoing higher risk surgeries. The guidelines state that "Preoperative resting 12-lead electrocardiogram (ECG) is reasonable for patients with known coronary heart disease, significant arrhythmia, peripheral arterial disease, cerebrovascular disease, or other significant structural heart disease." They give the strength of this recommendation a class IIa rating, which means that (1) the benefits largely outweigh the risks but additional studies with focused objectives are needed and (2) it is reasonable to perform procedure. The evidence on which this is based is rated B in quality. For patients who do not have known cardiac risk factors and are not undergoing low-risk surgery, the recommendations are more ambiguous and state "preoperative resting 12-lead ECG may be considered for asymptomatic patients without known coronary heart disease." This is given a weaker IIb recommendation based on B quality evidence.

To summarize the recommendations, those patients undergoing low-risk surgery do not require a preoperative ECG. When the surgery is not low-risk, patients with cardiovascular disease should get an ECG. For those who are neither high-risk patients nor getting a low-risk operation, ECG can be considered. The guidelines from the European Society of Cardiology and the European Society of Anaesthesiology are quite similar. They also recommend against routine ECGs in patients undergoing low-risk procedures but do recommend ECGs for patients with known cardiac risk factors undergoing surgeries other than low-risk with less firm recommendations for those patients who are less at risk. What differs from the ACC/AHA recommendations is that the European Society gives less weight to the evidence supporting the use of preoperative ECG for surgery that is not low-risk.

ROUTINE PREOPERATIVE COAGULATION STUDIES

The most common tests ordered preoperatively to assess bleeding risk are the prothrombin time (PT), partial thromboplastin time (PTT), and platelet count. It is uncommon to find true significant abnormalities of the PT and PTT,[9] and these tests should not be ordered in an unselected way. Although it may seem intuitive that an elevation in any of these tests would predict an increased risk of bleeding during surgery, there is no evidence that they have any value in predicting operative bleeding in a patient with no history of bleeding or liver disease. Taking an accurate bleeding history is much more important than unselected blood work. This history should consist of reviewing medications that might affect hemostasis and the patient's personal and family bleeding history. Most significant bleeding disorders will be picked up by an appropriate line of questioning. Bleeding disorders like hemophilia are rare and will likely be known to the physician long before the adult patient requires surgery.

Other bleeding disorders, such as von Willebrand disease, may not be revealed by routine coagulation studies and are more likely going to be discovered by taking a thorough bleeding history. When the history does reveal a personal or family history of unusual bleeding, further testing is indicated.

Patient undergoing neurosurgical procedures are at particularly high risk of bleeding complications; however, a study in the *Journal of Neurosurgery* suggests that coagulation studies have little power to predict complications for these high-risk patients.[10] In this 2012 analysis, the records of almost 12,000 neurosurgery patients in the 2006 to 2009 American College of Surgeons National Surgical Quality Improvement Program database were retrospectively reviewed. They found that more than 90% of patients had coagulation studies performed before neurosurgical procedures. Multivariate logistic regression models were then used to examine how accurately abnormalities in routine coagulation studies predicted the need for transfusion, return to the operating room, or 30-day mortality. Researchers found that the bleeding history was more predictive of bleeding complications and had a higher sensitivity for predicting those operative outcomes than did routine blood tests. The investigators concluded that routine coagulation studies should not be done in patients without a history of bleeding and further calculated that doing away with this testing before neurosurgery procedures would save more than 81 million dollars annually in the United States alone.

Even when the PT and PTT are abnormal, they do not necessarily predict an increased risk of bleeding. In a meta-analysis of 9 studies looking at the predictive value of preoperative coagulation studies, a committee of the British Haematology Society calculated the positive predictive value and likelihood ratios for an abnormal test predicting bleeding.[11] The positive predictive value for an abnormal clotting study to predict postoperative bleeding ranged from 0.03 to 0.22 with a likelihood ratio ranging from 0.99 to 5.10. Although the studies were not randomized, these numbers suggest that preoperative coagulation studies have little power to predict operative bleeding if used in unselected patients. Consequently, the British Committee for Standards in Haematology recommends against routine preoperative studies of bleeding.

SUMMARY

Given the low-risk nature of cataract surgery, no preoperative testing is indicated unless the patient needs such testing for another reason. Although ECGs may have a role in preoperative testing in patients who are at high risk of (or have) cardiovascular disease or if the procedure carries with it significant operative risks, they are often not necessary for many patients or procedures. In addition, urinalysis and coagulation studies should not routinely be obtained on patients before surgery because they have not been shown to have any value in predicting surgical complications. Although all of these tests are not expensive on an individual basis, the aggregate cost is substantial. As good stewards of the medical system, physicians need to use these tests more judiciously.

REFERENCES

1. Roizen MF. More preoperative assessment by physicians and less by laboratory tests. N Engl J Med 2000;342:204–5.
2. Schein OD. Assessing what we do: the example of preoperative medical testing. Arch Ophthalmol 1996;114:1129–31.

3. Chen CI. Preoperative medical testing in Medicare patients undergoing cataract surgery. N Engl J Med 2015;372:1530–8.
4. Schein OD, Katz J, Bass EB, et al. The value of routine preoperative testing before cataract surgery: study of medical testing for cataract surgery. N Engl J Med 2000;342:168–75.
5. Sousa R, Muñoz-Mahamud E, Quayle J, et al. Is asymptomatic bacteriuria a risk factor for prosthetic joint infection? Clin Infect Dis 2014;59(1):41–7.
6. Payne CJ, Payne AR, Gibson SC, et al. Is there still a role for preoperative 12-lead electrocardiography? World J Surg 2011;35:2611–6.
7. Jeger RV, Probst C, Arsenic R, et al. Long-term prognostic value of the preoperative 12-lead electrocardiogram before major noncardiac surgery in coronary artery disease. Am Heart J 2006;151:508–13.
8. Fleisher LA, Fleischmann KE, Auerbach AD, et al. 2014 ACC/AHA guideline on perioperative cardiovascular evaluation and management of patients undergoing non cardiac surgery: executive summary: a report of the American College of Cardiology/American Heart Association Task Force on Practice Guidelines. Circulation 2014;130:2215.
9. Bushick JB, Eisenberg JM, Kinman J, et al. Pursuit of abnormal coagulation screening tests generates modest hidden preoperative costs. J Gen Intern Med 1989;4:493.
10. Seicean A, Schiltz NK, Seicean S, et al. Use and Utility of Preoperative Hemostatic Screening and Patient History in Adult Neurosurgical Patients. J Neurosurg 2012 May;116(5):1097–105.
11. Chee YL, Crawford JC, Watson HG, et al. Guidelines on the assessment of bleeding risk prior to surgery or invasive procedures. British Committee for Standards in Haematology. Br J Haematol 2008;140:496.

The Cost-Effective Evaluation of Uncomplicated Headache

Marilyn Katz, MD

KEYWORDS

- Uncomplicated headache • Primary headache • Secondary headache
- Cost-effective

KEY POINTS

- Headache is a common ailment in the general population.
- Using the pneumonic SSNOOP can help identify red-flag features.
- If a red flag exists, workup will be focused on that particular sign or symptom.
- In the case of a primary or uncomplicated headache, no head imaging is warranted.

INTRODUCTION

Primary headache is head pain that is not attributable to an underlying etiology known to cause headaches and is considered somewhat a diagnosis of exclusion. The lifetime prevalence of headaches is 93% for men and 99% for women.[1] Head pain results in more than 4 million visits to the emergency room annually and accounts for 12 million visits to outpatient offices.[2] The direct health care costs of migraines, one subset of primary headaches, is estimated at $1 billion annually, whereas the indirect costs due to missed work days and missed function nears $13 billion annually.[3] It is estimated that there is $146 to $211 million spent annually on imaging for headaches.[4] Therefore, an evidence-based, cost-effective approach to the evaluation of patients presenting with a chief complaint of headache can have a significant impact on the annual cost of care.

PATHOPHYSIOLOGY AND CLASSIFICATION

The true pathophysiology of primary headaches is not well understood, but, by definition, is not attributable to an underlying disorder. The long-held belief that migraines were due to vascular dilation has sufficiently been disproved[5] and current research

Disclosure: Dr M. Katz reports no conflicts of interest.
Department of Medicine, University of Connecticut School of Medicine, 263 Farmington Avenue, Farmington, CT 06030, USA
E-mail address: mkatz@uchc.edu

Med Clin N Am 100 (2016) 1009–1017
http://dx.doi.org/10.1016/j.mcna.2016.04.009   medical.theclinics.com
0025-7125/16/$ – see front matter © 2016 Elsevier Inc. All rights reserved.

indicates a neurologic mechanism. In contrast, secondary headaches are due to an underlying etiology, so the mechanism through which they cause pain is dependent on that comorbidity. The International Headache Society (IHS) is the primary entity responsible for classification of headaches, and the most recent classification system is the International Classification of Headache Disorders, 2nd Edition (ICHD-2), although the International Classification of Headache Disorders, 3rd Edition beta (ICHD-III beta) is currently in progress.

Primary, or uncomplicated, headaches represent most headaches and primarily consist of migraine and tension headaches. Diagnosis is based on a constellation of symptoms elicited from the patient history, while simultaneously ruling out a secondary cause is also imperative. Combined, migraine and tension headaches comprise 90% of primary headache types. Migraine headaches affect approximately 18.2% of women and 6.5% of men,[6] with an overall 11.7% 1-year prevalence (17.1% for women and 5.6% for men).[7] Tension headaches have a lifetime prevalence of 88% of women and 69% of men.[1]

Migraine headaches are likely less prevalent than tension headaches in the population, but present more to the health care system for evaluation. They can occur with or without an aura. The following are criteria for migraine without aura[8]:

A. At least 5 attacks fulfilling criteria B to D
B. Headache attacks lasting 4 to 72 hours (untreated or unsuccessfully treated)
C. Headache has at least 2 of the following characteristics:
    a. Unilateral location
    b. Pulsating quality
    c. Moderate or severe pain intensity
    d. Aggravation by or causing avoidance of routine physical activity
D. During headache at least 1 of the following
    a. Nausea and/or vomiting
    b. Photophobia and phonophobia
E. Not attributed to another disorder

Tension-type headaches (TTH) are broken down into 4 subgroups: acute, episodic, chronic, and probable. The following are criteria for acute TTH[9]:

A. At least 10 episodes occurring on less than 1 day per month on average (<12 days per year) and fulfilling criteria B to D
B. Headache lasting from 30 minutes to 7 days
C. Headache has at least 2 of the following characteristics:
    a. Bilateral location
    b. Pressing/tightening (nonpulsating) quality
    c. Mild or moderate intensity
    d. Not aggravated by routine physical activity
D. Both of the following:
    a. No nausea or vomiting (anorexia may occur)
    b. No more than 1 of photophobia or phonophobia
E. Not attributed to another disorder

There are several variations of migraine and TTHs. Furthermore, there are additional primary headache syndromes that do not fit into these categories. **Table 1** outlines the primary headache syndromes, their variations, and corresponding International Classification of Diseases, 10th Revision (ICD-10) codes.

Unfortunately, headaches are not always benign, and can be secondary to an underlying problem that can cause significant harm if the diagnosis is missed. Although there

Table 1
IHS ICHD-II classification of primary headaches

Primary Headache Type	IHS	Headache Type	Notes	ICD 10
Migraine	1.1	Migraine without aura	—	G43.0
	1.2	Migraine with aura	—	G43.10x
	1.3	Childhood periodic syndromes that are commonly precursors of migraine	—	G43.82x
	1.4	Retinal migraine	Must exclude other causes of transient monocular blindness (amaurosis fugax) such as optic neuropathy or carotid dissection	G43.81
	1.5	Complications of migraine	—	G43.3
	1.6	Probable migraine	If missing one of the features needed to fulfil all criteria for above disorders	G43.83
Tension-Type Headache (TTH)	2.1	Infrequent episodic TTH	—	G44.2x
	2.2	Frequent episodic TTH	—	G44.2x
	2.3	Chronic TTH	—	G44.2x
	2.4	Probable TTH	—	G44.2x
Cluster headache and other trigeminal cephalalgias	3.1	Cluster headache	—	G44.0x
	3.2	Paroxysmal hemicrania	—	G44.0x
	3.3	Short-lasting unilateral neuralgiform headache attacks with conjunctival injection and tearing (SUNCT)	—	G44.08
	3.4	Probable trigeminal autonomic cephalgia	—	G44.08
Other primary headaches	4.1	Primary stabbing headache	—	G44.800
	4.2	Primary cough headache	Neuroimaging important to differentiate from secondary headache	G44.803
	4.3	Primary exertional headache	On first occurrence, mandatory to exclude subarachnoid hemorrhage and aortic dissection	G44.804
	4.4	Primary headache associated with sexual activity	On first occurrence of orgasmic headache, mandatory to exclude subarachnoid hemorrhage and aortic dissection	G44.805
	4.5	Hypnic headache	Must exclude intracranial disorders	G44.80
	4.6	Primary thunderclap headache	Must have normal LP and head imaging for diagnosis	G44.80
	4.7	Hemicrania continua	—	G44.80
	4.8	New daily-persistent headache (NDPH)	—	G44.2

Abbreviations: ICHD, International Classification of Headache Disorders; IHS, International Headache Society; LP, lumbar puncture.
   Adapted from Headache Classification Subcommittee of the International Headache Society. The International Classification of Headache Disorders. Cephalalgia 2004;24(suppl 1):1:160.

are many causes of secondary headaches, the diagnoses related to significant patient morbidity and mortality are listed in **Table 2**. Fear of these diagnoses often drives both physician and patient anxiety, which can result in unnecessary neuroimaging.

PATIENT HISTORY

Eliciting a thorough headache history is the most important first step in evaluating a patient with headache. The history really serves two main purposes. The first is to identify historical clues that may help characterize or diagnose the headache. The second is to rule out secondary (and often dangerous) causes of headache by identifying historical red flags. It is important to assess the location, duration, severity, onset, type of pain, associated symptoms, and aggravating and alleviating factors. It is also

Table 2
Underlying etiologies associated with red-flag symptoms

IHS	Headache Type	Features
6.1	Headache attributed to ischemic stroke or transient ischemic attack	Accompanied by focal neurologic signs and/or alterations in consciousness
6.2	Headache attributed to nontraumatic intracranial hemorrhage	6.2.2: Headache attributed to subarachnoid hemorrhage (SAH). Need neuroimaging (CT or MRI T2 or FLAIR) or CSF evidence of nontraumatic SAH with or without other clinical signs. Classic "thunderclap" headache.
6.4	Headache attributed to arteritis	6.4.1: Headache attributed to giant cell arteritis. Need tender temporal artery and elevated ESR or CRP or temporal artery biopsy
6.6	Headache attributed to cerebral venous thrombosis (CVT)	90% of cases associated with focal neurologic sign. Diagnosis with CT scan plus CT angiography or MRI plus MRA
7.1	Headache attributed to high cerebrospinal fluid pressure	7.1.1: Headache attributed to idiopathic intracranial hypertension
7.3	Headache attributed to noninfectious inflammatory disease	7.3.1: Headache attributed to neurosarcoidosis 7.3.2: Headache attributed to aseptic (noninfectious) meningitis
7.4	Headache attributed to intracranial neoplasm	—
9.1	Headache attributed to intracranial infection	Bacterial meningitis, lymphocytic meningitis, encephalitis, subdural empyema
9.2	Headache attributed to systemic infection	—
9.3	Headache attributed to HIV/AIDS	—
10.3	Headache attributed to arterial hypertension	Pheochromocytoma, hypertensive crisis with/without encephalopathy, preeclampsia, eclampsia, secondary to pressors

Abbreviations: CRP, C-reactive protein; CSF, cerebrospinal fluid; CT, computed tomography; ESR, erythrocyte sedimentation rate; FLAIR, fluid-attenuated inversion recovery; HIV, human immunodeficiency virus; MRA, magnetic resonance angiography.

Adapted from Headache Classification Subcommittee of the International Headache Society. The International Classification of Headache Disorders. Cephalalgia 2004;24(suppl 1):1:160.

important to assess precipitating factors, prior workup (eg, studies, treatments), and exertional features. The use of a headache diary can help identify patterns and triggers to both the patient and provider that may not be initially apparent. The pneumonic "SSNOOP" can be helpful in identifying red-flag features, see **Table 3**. There are numerous types of secondary headaches, but fewer that pose risk of harmful sequelae if undiagnosed. For that reason, we focus on red flags to differentiate a worrisome headache from one that will not cause any long-term effects. If no red flags are present, then the odds favor that one is dealing with a primary (uncomplicated) headache.

A headache history must include a thorough review of a patient's past medical, family, and social histories. This review may help identify conditions and diagnoses that are current to the patient but may also identify undiagnosed conditions. As an example, in an effort to rule out the possibility of a concomitant malignancy, it is important to elicit any personal history of cancer, determine if the individual is up to date on appropriate cancer screenings, and identify other risk factors for malignancy, such as family history or personal risk factors, such as smoking.

Medication history should include all prescription, over-the-counter (OTC), and herbal remedies. Initiation, termination, or chronic use of one or more agents may correlate to the headaches and their severity. Patients may not readily make this connection, so asking details about specific doses and frequencies is important.

Social history should include smoking, alcohol, recreational drugs, and caffeine usage at a minimum. In addition, a detailed sexual history may identify human immunodeficiency virus risk factors that could be important. Other considerations would be environmental and occupational exposures that could trigger the headaches or be a causative agent, and travel history may indicate an infectious etiology not native to where the patient is presenting with headache.

A full review of symptoms in addition to what was already discussed in the history of present illness may uncover clues to unrecognized ailments. Key systems would be constitutional (geared toward malignancy or infection), integumentary, ear nose and throat, and neurologic.

PHYSICAL EXAMINATION

The goal of the physical examination when evaluating the patient in the setting of uncomplicated headache is to rule out the possibility of a secondary headache. By

Table 3
Red flags: "SSNOOP"

Pneumonic	Red Flag
S	Systemic symptom (fever, weight loss)
S	Secondary risk factors (human immunodeficiency virus, systemic cancer)
N	Neurologic symptoms or abnormal signs (confusion, impaired alertness or consciousness)
O	Onset: sudden, abrupt, or split-second
O	Older: new-onset and progressive headache, especially in middle age >50 y (giant cell arteritis)
P	Previous headache history: first headache or different (change in attack frequency, severity or clinical features)

Data from Silberstein SD, Lipton RB, Dalessio DJ. Overview, diagnosis, and classification. In: Silberstein SD, Lipton RB, Dalessio DJ, editors. Wolff's headache and other head pain. 7th edition. Oxford (United Kingdom): Oxford University Press; 2001. p. 20.

definition, an uncomplicated headache would not be expected to have any positive findings on careful examination. Ironically, in a 2004 emergency department study by Locker and colleagues,[10] it was determined that this step was lacking in many emergency room visits. This could be one driver of unnecessary neuroimaging.

In the examination, it is important to note the general appearance of the patient. Does the patient appear well or are there signs of cachexia? Are there clues to suggest thyroid dysfunction (eg, goiter, proptosis) or infection? Vital signs, especially temperature, heart rate, and blood pressure are particularly useful, but respiratory rate may indicate an issue with intracranial pressure or infectious agent, and body mass index may increase the risk of idiopathic intracranial hypertension (formerly known as pseudotumor cerebri). A thorough skin examination is needed to rule out any rashes. An evaluation of the temporomandibular (TMJ) joint and teeth (to look for signs of excessive attrition) are done to rule out TMJ dysfunction. In addition, a thorough neurologic examination is needed that includes assessments of mental status, cranial nerves, motor strength, sensory or coordination deficits, and a fundu-scopic examination.

IMAGING AND ADDITIONAL TESTING

Making the determination between primary and secondary headaches is the most important determination, as secondary headaches carry significant morbidity and mortality. A study by Mert and colleagues[11] determined that unilaterality and a spec-ified trigger increased the risk of primary headaches by 1.431 and 1.440, respectively, whereas a comorbid medical condition increased the risk of a secondary headache by 4.643.

Over the past 2 decades, there have been numerous studies and evidence-based recommendations to support empiric treatment without the need for neuro-imaging in these cases. This has been recently reinforced through the Choosing Wisely Campaign (**Tables 4** and **5**). Patients should be educated on what signs and symp-toms to look for should something change and provided instructions of what to do. Close follow-up with the patients is recommended in case there is a change to the headache pattern or treatment is not effective.

Sempere and colleagues[12] determined that the pretest probability for a significant intracranial finding in a chronic headache (lasting at least 4 weeks) with a normal neurologic examination was 0.9% (95% confidence interval 0.5–1.4), whereas the overall risk of a significant finding was 1.2% and an insignificant finding 0.75%. You

Table 4 Choosing wisely recommendations regarding the diagnosis of headaches	
Society	**Recommendation**
American Headache Society	Don't perform computed tomography (CT) imaging for headache when MRI is available, except in emergency settings.
American Headache Society	Don't perform neuroimaging studies in patients with stable headaches that meet criteria for migraine.
American College of Radiology	Don't do imaging for uncomplicated headache.
American Academy of Neurology	Don't perform electroencephalography (EEG) for headaches.

Data from Choosing Wisely: An initiative of the ABIM Foundation. Clinician lists. Available at: http://www.choosingwisely.org/clinician-lists/. Accessed April 26, 2016.

Table 5	
Choosing wisely recommendations regarding the management of headaches	
Society	Recommendation
American Headache Society	Don't recommend prolonged or frequent use of over-the-counter (OTC) pain medications for headache.
American Headache Society	Don't prescribe opioid or butalbital-containing medications as first-line treatment for recurrent headache disorders.
American Academy of Neurology	Don't use opioid or butalbital treatment for migraine except as a last resort.
American Headache Society	Don't recommend surgical deactivation of migraine trigger points outside of a clinical trial.

Data from Choosing Wisely: An initiative of the ABIM Foundation. Clinician lists. Available at: http://www.choosingwisely.org/clinician-lists/. Accessed April 26, 2016.

and colleagues[13] determined that only 2% of computed tomography (CT) and 5% of MRI scans performed for headaches revealed treatable intracranial pathology.

Based on the US Health Consortium recommendations, the data were insufficient to make evidence-based recommendations on MRI versus CT in the evaluation of migraine or other nonacute headache (Grade C).[14] However, the American Headache Society recommends against CT when MRI is available (see **Table 4**).

In the setting of the emergency department, a noncontrast CT scan is often performed first due to speed, convenience, and a frequent need to rule out a hemorrhage. If intravenous contrast is given before either CT or MRI and indeed a hemorrhage does exist, the contrast will mix with the hemorrhaged blood and make it difficult to differentiate structures. CT uses ionizing radiation to construct 3-dimensional images from compiling high-resolution anatomic cross sections. MRI uses magnetic fields to construct images and has an enhanced ability to distinguish soft tissue versus CT. MRIs take much longer than CTs and show much more detail and are not as readily available.

Both imaging modalities run the risk of uncovering incidental abnormalities. One study of 1000 asymptomatic volunteers undergoing neuroimaging demonstrated significant findings in 0.6%[15] of participants, whereas a study of 3672 patients undergoing neuroimaging for stroke found the rate of findings not attributable to stroke to be 1.1%.[16]

For patients with frequent and severe headaches, despite appropriate counseling and medication therapies, their anxiety regarding a potential secondary cause of their headache may still exist. Howard and colleagues[17] investigated whether or not neuroimaging actually reduced patient anxiety and worry, but the results were ultimately inconclusive. However, this study also showed that providing patients with scores greater than 11 on the Hospital Anxiety and Depression Score actually decreased overall costs to the health care system ($P = .03$). In such patients, it may be reasonable to perform neuroimaging to alleviate patient fears.[18]

MANAGEMENT

Based on the evidence to date, for patients with a normal physical examination, who meet criteria for primary headache syndrome and no red flags are identified, neuroimaging is not necessary. Empiric treatment for presumed uncomplicated headache syndrome is recommended. If the patient does not clearly meet criteria for a primary headache syndrome but does not have any red flags or physical examination findings, prescribing the use of a headache diary is an appropriate next step to help aid in diagnosis. At the same time, medications can be used to treat any discomfort the patient is experiencing.

If a red flag exists, further workup through laboratory studies and/or neuroimaging would be appropriate based on the nature of the finding. For instance, if the patient has unilateral temporal pain and jaw claudication, an erythrocyte sedimentation rate and temporal artery biopsy would be the appropriate next step toward a diagnosis of giant cell arteritis, although the patient with a thunderclap headache would need a noncontrast CT followed by a lumbar puncture to rule out subarachnoid hemorrhage.

REFERENCES

1. Rasmussen BK, Jensen R, Schroll M, et al. Epidemiology of headache in a general population—a prevalence study. J Clin Epidemiol 1991;44:1147–57.
2. Smitherman TA, Burch R, Sheikh H, et al. The prevalence, impact, and treatment of migraine and severe headaches in the United States: a review of statistics from national surveillance studies. Headache 2013;53(3):427–36.
3. Hu X, Markson LE, Lipton RB, et al. Burden of migraine in the United States: disability and economic costs. Arch Intern Med 1999;159(8):813–8.
4. Schwartz AL, Landon BE, Elshaug AG, et al. Measuring low-value care in Medicare. JAMA Intern Med 2014;174(7):1067–76.
5. Amin FM, Asghar MS, Anders H, et al. Magnetic resonance angiography of intracranial and extracranial arteries in patients with spontaneous migraine without aura: a cross sectional study. Lancet Neurol 2013;12:454–61.
6. Lipton RB, Stewart WF, Diamond S, et al. Prevalence and burden of migraine in the United States: data from the American Migraine Study II. Headache 2001; 41:646–57.
7. Lipton RB, Bigal ME, Diamond M, et al. Migraine prevalence, disease burden, and the need for preventive therapy. Neurology 2007;68(5):343–9.
8. Available at: http://ihs-classification.org/en/02_klassifikation/02_teil1/01.01.00_migraine.html. Accessed November 30, 2015.
9. Available at: http://ihs-classification.org/en/02_klassifikation/02_teil1/02.01.00_tension.html. Accessed November 30, 2015.
10. Locker T, Mason S, Rigby A. Headache management—are we doing enough? An observational study of patients presenting with headache to the emergency department. Emerg Med J 2004;21(3):327–32.
11. Mert E, Özge A, Taşdelen B, et al. What clues are available for differential diagnosis of headaches in emergency settings? J Headache Pain 2008;9(2):89–97.
12. Sempere AP, Porta-Etessam J, Medrano V, et al. Neuroimaging in the evaluation of patients with non-acute headache. Cephalalgia 2004;25(1):30–5.
13. You JJ, Purdy I, Rothwell DM, et al. Indications for and results of outpatient computed tomography and magnetic resonance imaging in Ontario. Can Assoc Radiol J 2008;59(3):135–43.
14. Frishberg BM, Rosenberg JH, Matchar DB, et al. Evidence-based guidelines in the primary care setting: neuroimaging in patients with nonacute headache. Am Acad Neurol 2000. Available at: https://protocols.xray.ufl.edu/live_protocols/documents/guidance/UF/headache_guide.pdf.
15. Katzman GL, Dagher AP, Patronas NJ. Incidental findings on brain magnetic resonance imaging from 1000 asymptomatic volunteers. JAMA 1999;282:36–9.

16. Yue NC, Longstreth WT Jr, Elster AD, et al. Clinically serious abnormalities found incidentally at MR imaging of the brain: data from the Cardiovascular Health Study. Radiology 1997;202:41–6.
17. Howard L, Wessely S, Leese M, et al. Are investigations anxiolytic or anxiogenic? A randomised controlled trial of neuroimaging to provide reassurance in chronic daily headache. J Neurol Neurosurg Psychiatry 2005;76(11):1558–64.
18. Practice parameter. Evidence-based guidelines for migraine headache (an evidence-based review). Neurology 2000;55(6):754–62.

The Cost-Effective Evaluation of Syncope

Steven Angus, MD

KEYWORDS

- Syncope • Classification • Cost-effective • Risk-stratification

KEY POINTS

- Syncope is a common occurrence with a lifetime incidence of 40% and leads to a significant cost-burden on the US health system.
- A meticulous history and physical examination, including orthostatics and electrocardiogram, are the most cost-effective tools in diagnosing syncope.
- Routine blood tests, neuroimaging with computed tomography scans, MRIs, carotid Doppler, echocardiography, and inpatient telemetry monitoring rarely contribute to the diagnosis but add substantial cost.
- There are multiple risk stratification tools that help identify high-risk patients and guide management.
- Applying these tools can reduce syncope-related costs substantially without increasing risks to patients.

INTRODUCTION

Syncope is defined as the transient loss of consciousness associated with the inability to maintain postural tone.[1] Cohort studies suggested a lifetime prevalence of 40% in the adult population, though the exact incidence is difficult to define because many patients with syncope do not seek medical attention. The incidence is higher with advancing age, potentially related to an increase in prescription of vasoactive drugs and increasing incidence of cardiac arrhythmias in the elderly population.[2]

Studies estimated that syncope accounts for 3% of all the emergency department visits and that approximately one-third of these visits result in hospitalization.[1,3] Thus, syncope accounts for anywhere from between 1% to 6% of all hospital admissions.[1]

Data from 2001 through 2010 show that the proportion of patients presenting to the emergency department with syncope and then admitted to the hospital has remained stable despite the publication of multiple clinical guidelines and strategies for optimizing resource utilization in the emergency department.[3] More worrisome, the rate

Disclosure: Dr S. Angus reports no conflicts of interest.
Department of Medicine, University of Connecticut School of Medicine, 263 Farmington Avenue, Farmington, CT 06030, USA
E-mail address: angus@uchc.edu

Med Clin N Am 100 (2016) 1019–1032
http://dx.doi.org/10.1016/j.mcna.2016.04.010
0025-7125/16/$ – see front matter © 2016 Elsevier Inc. All rights reserved.

medical.theclinics.com

of utilization of advanced imaging for syncope patients has increased significantly from 20% to 45% over this same time frame.[3]

Syncope has a considerable direct and indirect socioeconomic burden. The cost of syncope remains quite substantial with the in-hospital expenses making up most of these costs. The estimated costs for syncope-related hospitalizations in 2000 approached $2.5 billion and were driven the high admission rate and by testing. Despite the development of tools for risk stratifying patients presenting with syncope, many patients continue to be admitted at an estimated cost of $5400 per admission.[4] Considering that admission and additional inpatient workup rarely leads to a more specific cause of syncope, it has been estimated that the average cost per clear etiologic diagnosis of syncope approaches $78,000.[4]

PATHOPHYSIOLOGY OR CLASSIFICATION

Syncope is secondary to a brief decrease in cerebral blood flow that spontaneously and completely resolves and requires no resuscitation.[1] In most cases, diminished cerebral perfusion is caused by a transient decrease in systemic blood pressure.[5,6] Mechanistically, systemic blood pressure is determined by cardiac output and peripheral vascular resistance, and a decrease in either can cause syncope. More often than not, a combination of both mechanisms is present.

The causes of transient low cardiac output include reflex bradycardia, cardiac arrhythmias, structural heart disease, and inadequate venous return due to volume depletion or venous pooling.[6] Decreased peripheral vascular resistance may be caused by primary or secondary impairments in the autonomic nervous system.

Classification of syncope based on pathophysiologic mechanisms allows for grouping of entities with common presentations based on the cause of the drop in systemic blood pressure (**Table 1**). Syncope is typically classified into neurally mediated syncope (including vasovagal syncope, carotid sinus hypersensitivity, and situational syncope), orthostatic syncope, and cardiac syncope. Neurally mediated syncope is the most common form of syncope when all age groups are considered; it is a particularly common cause of syncope in young healthy adults without a history of structural cardiac disease. Vasovagal syncope has a lifetime incidence of 20% in the general population.[1,6] It is often seen in young, otherwise healthy patients but may occur in all age groups.

Table 1
Classification and basic pathophysiologic mechanism of syncope

Type	Pathophysiology	Subtypes
Neurally Mediated (reflex)	Inappropriate increase in sympathetic or parasympathetic tone leading to vasodepressor symptoms (hypotension), cardioinhibitory symptoms (bradycardia), or both	Vasovagal Carotid sinus syndrome Situational syncope
Cardiac	Decreased cardiac output	Arrhythmia Structural heart disease Ischemia
Orthostatic Hypotension	Insufficient vasoconstriction in response to orthostatic stress (standing)	Primary autonomic failure Secondary autonomic failure Drug-induced Volume depletion

Syncope caused by carotid sinus hypersensitivity tends to occur in older men and may be associated with concurrent atherosclerotic disease. This form of syncope seems to occur in close relationship with mechanical manipulation of the neck, during shaving, or from tight neck collars. Situational syncope includes a wide range of clinical scenarios in which syncope closely follows a trigger and includes entities such as cough syncope, postmicturition syncope, defecation syncope, and so forth.

Orthostatic hypotension should be diagnosed as the cause of syncope when there is documentation of posturally induced hypotension associated with syncope or presyncope. The classic form of orthostatic hypotension is defined by a decline in systolic blood pressure of at least 20 mm Hg after 3 to 5 minutes of assuming a standing posture. Volume depletion, medications, and certain endocrinopathies may lead to orthostatic hypotension, as can primary neurologic disorders such as Parkinson disease.

Cardiac causes of syncope include arrhythmias and structural heart disease. Both tachycardia and bradycardia may lead to syncope. Ventricular tachycardia is an important cause of syncope to consider in patients with known structural heart disease. Supraventricular tachycardia during atrial flutter or atrial fibrillation may be associated with syncope at the onset of an episode before vascular compensation occurs. Bradycardia arrhythmias that may lead to syncope include those induced by sinus node dysfunction (sinus pauses, sinoatrial bradycardia), as well as by high-degree atrioventricular (AV) blocks (Mobitz type II second-degree heart block or third-degree AV block). When seen on EKG, these entities can be considered diagnostic of a bradycardia-induced syncope.

Structural cardiac causes of syncope include hypertrophic cardiomyopathy, aortic stenosis, and acute myocardial infarction. Syncope may be related to the reduced cardiac output in these entities in conjunction with a neurally mediated reflex vasodilatation. Decreased cardiac output in the setting of structural heart disease may be worsened by tachyarrhythmias by precluding adequate venous filling of the ventricle, thus leading to syncope by this additional mechanism.[6]

THE HISTORY AND PHYSICAL EXAMINATION

A complete history and comprehensive physical examination is the most cost-effective means of diagnosing syncope.[6,7] A detailed history and physical examination, plus a 12-lead electrocardiogram (ECG), lead to initial diagnosis in upwards of two-thirds of cases, with a diagnostic accuracy as high as 88%.[1,2] It is estimated that up to 80% of the identifiable causes of syncope are determined in the emergency department,[1] thus admission for further diagnostic testing is infrequently warranted.

THE HISTORY

A complete history is important for differentiating syncopal from nonsyncopal causes of loss of consciousness and to differentiate patients at risk of cardiac syncope from other noncardiac causes. Typical syncope is brief, with complete loss of consciousness lasting 20 seconds or less. When the duration of loss of consciousness is longer, the differentiation between syncope and other causes of loss of consciousness can be difficult.[6] Cardiac syncope carries a high mortality in all age groups, with the Framingham study showing a hazard ratio for death of 2.4 for patients with cardiac syncope compared with 1.17 for patients with vasovagal syncope and orthostatic hypotension over a follow-up period of 8.5 years,[2] thus illustrating the importance of identifying this group of patients.

Multiple factors should be taken into account when eliciting a history from the patient who has experienced syncope. Key historical elements that may help the clinician determine the cause of syncope may be ascertained by asking about the events leading up to the event, the presence of a prodrome, events that happened during the event based on eye-witness accounts, and symptoms during recovery (**Table 2**).[2] Some forms of syncope may be preceded by a prodromal phase in which various symptoms, such as lightheadedness, nausea, sweating, weakness, or visual disturbances, herald that syncope is imminent. The patient's age must also be considered because the frequency with which different disorders cause syncope is age-dependent: cardiac syncope, which is often more serious, is rare in younger people but accounts for one-third of syncopal events in older patients.[2]

Table 2
Key historical elements in the evaluation of syncope

Key Questions to Ask all Syncope Patients	Type of Syncope to Consider
What happened just before the event (precipitants)	
Change in position from sitting to standing	Orthostasis
Sense of fear, pain, emotional situation	Vasovagal
Turning of head or shaving	Carotid sinus syndrome
Urination, defecation, coughing, swallowing	Situational syncope
Exercise	Cardiac
Prolonged standing	Orthostasis or vasovagal
Lying supine	Cardiac arrhythmia
No clear precipitant	Cardiac or vasovagal in elderly
Were there any symptoms before event (prodrome)	
Feeling warm, sweaty, or nauseous	Vasovagal
Lightheadedness, blurred vision, diming of vision	Orthostasis or vasovagal
Chest pain or dyspnea	Cardiac
Palpitations	Cardiac, specifically arrhythmia
What did people notice during the event	
Flaccid, loss of tone with minor twitching or myoclonic jerks	Suggests syncope
Rigid, posturing, rhythmic jerking	Suggests nonsyncopal cause (seizure)
Pallor, sweating	Suggests syncope
Cyanotic, "blue" color	Suggests nonsyncopal cause (seizure)
Eyes open, rolling back	Syncope or seizure
Eyes closed	Pseudoseizure, psychogenic syncope
Incontinence	Seizure but may be seen in syncope
Tongue biting	Suggests nonsyncopal cause (seizure)
How did patient feel after the event (recovery)	
Immediate and complete recovery	Syncope from any cause, arrhythmia
Nausea, vomiting, fatigue	Vasovagal
Prolonged confusion	Suggests nonsyncopal cause (seizure)
Transient disorientation	Neurally mediated syncope
Amnesia for the event	Neurally mediated syncope, particularly in elderly

A complete past medical history with a particular focus on pre-existing cardiac disease, diabetes, neurologic syndromes, and alcohol dependence should be obtained in all patients presenting with syncope. An accurate medication history, including over-the-counter medications, should also be obtained. Special attention should be paid to any recent changes in medications or dosages, with a particular focus on those medications known to lead to orthostatic hypotension (eg, antihypertensives, antidepressants, or those with anticholinergic side effects). A detailed family history should include questions about sudden cardiac death in family members because this factor has been shown to be significantly associated with a cardiac cause of syncope.[8] A history of dyspnea, chest pain, or palpitations also argues for a primary cardiac cause, particularly among patients who described a sensation of rapid and regular pulsations in the neck, which can be typical of AV nodal reentry tachycardia.[8]

THE PHYSICAL EXAMINATION

A complete and thorough physical examination should be done on all patients presenting with syncope. This will help elucidate the cause of the syncope but also serves to identify any traumatic consequences that may have occurred as a result of the syncope. Vital signs looking for bradycardia or tachycardia, tachypnea, and hypotension are an essential first step. All patients with syncope should have orthostatic vital signs measured and documented. A careful cardiac examination is warranted with particular focus on signs of aortic stenosis (an absent aortic component of the S2, a late peaking systolic ejection murmur, delayed carotid upstrokes, and a sustained apical impulse). One must also carefully differentiate between the murmur of aortic stenosis and hypertrophic cardiomyopathy, if present. A careful neurologic examination must also be performed; by definition, the neurologic examination result in syncope is normal. Any abnormal findings should lead the physician to consider a nonsyncopal event, such as an acute stroke or profound toxic or metabolic insult.[1] A thorough examination of the entire body is essential to detect trauma resulting from a fall.[1] Carotid sinus massage may also be considered in patients in whom carotid sinus sensitivity is suspected by history. **Table 3** reviews the European Society of Cardiology's recommendations for performing a carotid sinus massage. The

Table 3
Recommendations: carotid sinus massage

Recommendations	Class[a]	Level[b]
Indications		
CSM is indicated in patients >40 y with syncope of unknown cause after initial evaluation	I	B
CSM should be avoided in patients with previous TIA or stroke within the past 3 mo and in patients with carotid bruits (except if carotid Doppler studies excluded significant stenosis)	III	C
Diagnostic criteria		
CSM is diagnostic if syncope is reproduced in the presence of asystole longer than 3 s and/or a fall in systolic blood pressure >50 mm Hg	I	B

[a] Class of recommendation.
[b] Level of evidence.

Data from Moya A, Sutton R, Ammirati F, et al. Task force for the diagnosis and management of syncope, European Society of Cardiology (ESC), European Heart Rhythm Association (EHRA), Heart Failure Association (HFA), Heart Rhythm Society (HRS). Guidelines for the diagnosis and management of syncope (version 2009). Eur Heart J 2009;30(21):2646.

diagnosis of carotid sinus syncope requires reproduction of spontaneous symptoms during a 10-second sequential right and left carotid sinus massage while under continuous monitoring of heart rate and blood pressure. Performing this in the upright position is important because 30% of patients have the abnormal reflex only in the upright position.[6] Of note, the recommendation states that carotid sinus massage should be avoided in patients with previous transient ischemic attack (TIA), stroke within the past 3 months, or in those with carotid bruits (unless significant stenosis has been excluded by imaging).

INITIAL DIAGNOSTIC TESTING

After obtaining a complete history and conducting a thorough physical examination, including measurement of orthostatic vital signs, the cause of syncope may be evident in up to 60% of patients. If the cause of syncope is not evident, additional diagnostic testing is warranted but in a limited and symptom-directed fashion.

Electrocardiogram

Many societies, guidelines, and publications suggest that all patients presenting with syncope should have an ECG. The American College of Emergency Physicians clinical policy on syncope strongly recommends that an ECG be obtained in the initial evaluation of patients with syncope. They conclude that this is a rapid, inexpensive test and may identify the cause of syncope in 5% to 7% of cases.[1,9] Significant ECG findings that may suggest potential causes of syncope include evidence of acute coronary syndrome, severe bradycardia or tachycardia, prolonged QTC and QRS intervals, ventricular hypertrophy, or other pre-excitation conduction disturbances. The 2009 European Society of Cardiology guidelines identify certain ECG findings that are diagnostic of arrhythmia-induced syncope, including persistent sinus bradycardia (<40 beats/minute) in an awake patient, sinus pauses greater than 3 seconds or repetitive sinoatrial blocks, Mobitz II second-degree or third-degree heart blocks, alternating left and right bundle branch blocks, ventricular tachycardia or rapid supraventricular tachycardia, or evidence of pacemaker or implantable cardioverter-defibrillator malfunction with pauses.[6]

Blood Work

Routine laboratory screening in patients with syncope is not supported by clinical evidence nor is it cost-effective because it rarely aids in making a diagnosis or managing these patients.[1] The European syncope guidelines do not consider routine laboratory testing to be appropriate for syncope evaluation in all patients.[6] The American College of Physician's position paper reinforces that routine use of basic laboratory tests is not recommended for all patients but should be done if there are specific causes suspected based on the history and physical (eg, checking hemoglobin or hematocrit if profound blood loss or hypovolemia is thought to be the cause of syncope).[9]

Specific Laboratory Tests

The effectiveness of specialized testing, including D dimer, troponin, and brain natriuretic peptide (BNP), has been studied in syncope. None are recommended as cost-effective for routine measurement in all cases. Routine measurement of D dimers in patients presenting with syncope is not helpful in identifying either the cause of syncope or for use as a prognostic indicator. D-dimer testing should be reserved only for those patients in whom pulmonary embolism is suspected.[10] Measurement of troponin on a routine basis in patients presenting with syncope is also of limited effectiveness. Measurement of troponin should be reserved for those patients in whom acute coronary syndrome is suspected.[10] It has been observed that BNP levels have been increased in arrhythmias, thus raising interest in using BNP as biomarker of arrhythmogenic syncope.[10] The Risk stratification Of Syncope in the Emergency department (ROSE) rule (see later discussion) proposes using plasma BNP level to help in risk stratification by predicting serious cardiovascular outcomes and death; however, further validation of the prediction rule is warranted, as well as its utility in the evaluation of syncope.[11]

IMAGING AND ADDITIONAL DIAGNOSTIC TESTING
Testing in General

Routine imaging and additional testing adds to the cost of syncope while seemingly adding little to diagnostic accuracy. In an observational study of more than 2000 adults older than 65 years, cardiac enzymes, electroencephalogram (EEG), computed tomography (CT) of the head, and carotid ultrasonography helped to determine the cause of syncope in less than 1% of cases. In comparison, measurement of orthostatic vital signs contributed to the diagnosis 20% of the time at a fraction of the cost.[8] Neurologic studies, such as EEG, carotid Doppler, MRI, or CT scanning of the head, are almost never of use in the diagnosis of syncope. The latter modalities should be restricted to cases in which head injury may have occurred as a result of the collapse.[5]

It has also been suggested that routine echocardiography in patients with no evidence of structural heart disease is not useful and should be avoided.[2]

Computed Tomography or MRI

There is no current evidence that a patient with syncope benefits from routine neuroimaging. Head CT and MRI are generally of low yield and are overutilized in evaluation of patients with syncope. Patients who spontaneously and completely recover without treatment are unlikely to have structural brain abnormalities that would be seen on neuroimaging. Despite this, data in the National Hospital Ambulatory Medical Care Survey database revealed that the rate of advanced neuroimaging (CT or MRI) in the emergency department increased more than threefold from 2001 through 2010.[3] In patients whom the history or physical examination suggests a neurologic diagnosis other than syncope, imaging may be required.[1]

Echocardiography

Echocardiography is indicated for diagnosis and risk stratification in patients suspected of having structural heart disease (eg, hypertrophic cardiomyopathy or severe aortic stenosis) as the cause of their syncope.[1,2] Echocardiography is also useful in detecting the presence of other valvular abnormalities, wall motion abnormalities, elevated pulmonary pressures, and pericardial effusion.[1] Echocardiography has been shown to have the highest diagnostic yield in patients with a history of cardiac disease or in those who have abnormal ECG findings.[6] The current literature does not support as cost-effective the routine use of echocardiography as a screening test in patients with an otherwise negative screening evaluation (ie, no ECG abnormalities or evidence of structural heart disease by history or examination).[12]

Tilt Table Testing

Tilt table testing is used to evaluate patients with suspected neurally mediated syncope. It serves to reproduce those situations that may trigger overly robust neurally mediated reflexes. The pooling of blood and a decrease in venous return due to orthostatic stress and immobilization triggers this reflex, resulting in hypotension, usually associated with a decrease in heart rate. The exaggerated response is related to impaired vasoconstrictor capability followed by sympathetic withdrawal and vagal over activity.[6] Although it can be a helpful modality in certain circumstances, tilt testing is not needed in patients whose reflex syncope is readily diagnosed by clinical history or in patients with single or very infrequent episodes of syncope.[6]

To carefully monitor patients, the upright tilt table test is typically performed in an electrophysiology laboratory using continuous ECG and noninvasive blood pressure, looking for a pronounced cardioinhibitory response identified by symptomatic hypotension, bradycardia, or both.

The patient is first monitored in the supine position. Baseline heart rate and blood pressure measurements are obtained after 5 minutes in this position. The patient is then positioned in a head-up tilt position at an angle between 60° and 70° (based on the 2009 European Society of Cardiology guidelines).[6]

Patients are observed for 20 to 45 minutes with continuous ECG recording and heart rate, and patient symptoms are recorded at intervals of 3 to 5 minutes. The blood pressure should be monitored noninvasively by either beat-to-beat finger arterial monitoring or by arm cuff every 3 to 5 minutes. If the patient experiences loss of consciousness or a significant decrease in blood pressure, or heart rate associated with loss of the ability to maintain posture, the test is considered positive. If, after a period of 20 to 45 minutes, no symptoms have developed, the patient is returned to the supine position. A repeat head-up tilt portion while infusing isoproterenol to increase the heart rate 20% to 25% above the supine baseline is often used in these asymptomatic patients. Infusing isoproterenol induces more often than the standard test but also lowers the specificity of the test.[6]

Carotid Doppler

Guidelines currently recommend against neurovascular testing in cases of syncope because no studies have found value using them in patients with typical syncope.[6] In general, carotid artery duplex ultrasonography is a low-yield diagnostic test for diagnosing the cause of syncope.[13] Carotid artery duplex ultrasound may identify patients with asymptomatic atherosclerosis who would benefit from optimizing medical therapy but rarely aids in the diagnosis of syncope. In a small retrospective study, abnormalities were detected in 2% of patients but were not considered to be the primary cause of syncope.[8,14]

Continuous Electrocardiogram Monitoring

The gold standard for diagnosing arrhythmic syncope is correlating a documented arrhythmia with a patient's symptoms.[6] As a general rule, continuous ECG monitoring is indicated in syncope only when there is a high pretest probability of identifying arrhythmia. Clinical or resting ECG features that may suggest arrhythmic syncope include

- Syncope during exertion or while supine
- Palpitations at the time of syncope
- Family history of sudden cardiac death
- Nonsustained ventricular tachycardia
- Bifascicular block
- Prolonged or shortened QT interval

- Right bundle branch block pattern with ST elevation in leads V1 through V3 (typical of the Brugada pattern)
- Negative T waves in the right precordial leads and ventricular late potentials (suggestive of arrhythmogenic right ventricular cardiomyopathy).[6]

In these patients, it is reasonable to undertake continuous ECG monitoring using one of several methods.

Inpatient Telemetry Monitors

Inpatient telemetry monitoring is warranted only when the patient is at high risk for a life-threatening arrhythmia. Even when the high-risk findings listed previously are present, the diagnostic yield of ECG monitoring is still relatively low, approximating 15%.[6] Despite the low yield, guidelines suggest that the cost incurred by inpatient admission and telemetry monitoring in this high-risk population is warranted.[6]

Holter Monitor

Discharging patients with conventional 24-hour to 48-hour Holter recorders is inexpensive in terms of application but expensive in terms of cost per diagnosis. In most patients, symptoms do not recur during the monitoring. Thus, the true yield of a Holter monitor is as low as 1% to 2% in the general population.[6] It has been suggested that use of Holter monitoring may be more cost-effective in patients who have daily symptoms. In this context, a true negative Holter is very useful.[4] In a study looking at the usefulness of the 24-hour Holter monitor in patients with unexplained syncope, the diagnostic yield of Holter monitoring could be increased twofold when used in high-risk patients, those with a cardiac history and/or an abnormal ECG. Thus, in a carefully selected group of patients, yield of Holter monitor may be as high as 12%, and may be cost-effective, precluding additional testing.[15]

Loop or Event Recorders

External loop recorders are devices that continuously record and delete ECG tracings. When activated by the patient, typically during or after symptoms, 5 to 15 minutes of ECG recordings before, during, and after the symptoms are stored for analysis.[6] Studies have found that external loop recorders have an increased diagnostic yield and are more cost-effective than Holter monitoring.[4,16,17] Patient noncompliance with monitoring for more than a few weeks makes external loop recorders less cost-effective when syncope recurrence is quite infrequent.[4] Another study suggests that patient with infrequent episodes of syncope (2 in 6 months) should first undergo a tilt table test. A negative tilt table test carries a good outcome and may obviate an external loop recorder.[18]

Implantable loop recorders (ILRs) are small devices implanted subcutaneously. Although there are several disadvantages of using ILRs, including the high initial cost due to the need for a minor surgical procedure and the cost of the device itself, it has been suggested that using early implantation of ILRs may be more cost-effective than a strategy using conventional investigation, particularly when episodes are frequent and in those whom arrhythmic syncope is suspected but who are not deemed high-risk. Current guidelines recommend early use of ILRs in patients with unexplained syncope, when there are either recurrent symptoms or the suspicion for an arrhythmic cause is high.[6,19] In 2 randomized trials, a conventional strategy consisting of external loop recorders, tilt testing, and electrophysiologic study was used either before or after monitoring with an ILR. The diagnostic yield was similar in both groups but costs were reduced in the early ILR groups ($5875 per diagnosis vs $7891 per diagnosis).[4,20,21]

The Place of Reveal In the Care Pathway and Treatment of Patients with Unexplained Recurrent Syncope (PICTURE) registry also demonstrated the high yield and cost-effectiveness of early ILRs by highlighting the large number of diagnostic tests and referrals to specialists that patients in the conventional group underwent before ILR, adding to the cost without increasing diagnostic yield.[22]

RISK STRATIFICATION

The diagnostic evaluation of syncope in the outpatient or emergency room setting is often unstructured and not driven by the initial evaluation. Several studies have suggested that this unstructured approach leads to both excessive and unnecessary testing.[23,24] Several risk-stratification tools are available to help identify high-risk patients and guide the evaluation of syncope. Such tools serve to limit wasteful spending and prevent unnecessary admissions, the 2 largest drivers of cost in syncope. Some of these tools include the ROSE rule, Boston Syncope Rule, the San Francisco Syncope Rule, Osservatorio Epidemiologico sulla Sincope nel Lazio (OESIL) score, and the Evaluation of Guidelines in Syncope Study (EGSYS) score.[15,25–27] Although large-scale validation of these tools is pending, they all seem to have excellent sensitivity, good specificity, and excellent negative predictive value in identifying patients at high risk of mortality (**Table 4**). Strict adherence to the Boston rule would have decreased hospital admission by nearly 50% in this study population. Although these tools allow for excellent risk stratification, emergency room physicians often make disposition decisions that are not congruent with

Table 4
Scoring systems for stratifying risk after an episode of syncope

Score	San Francisco Syncope Rule	Rose Risk Score	OESIL Risk Score	EGSYS Syncope Score
Outcome Measures	Risk of serious outcome or death at 1 mo	Risk of serious outcome or death at 1 mo	Risk of all-cause mortality at 12 mo	Death from any cause
Risk Factors	Systolic blood pressure <90 mm Hg Shortness of breath ECG: nonsinus rhythm or new changes present History of congestive heart failure Hematocrit <30%	Brain natriuretic peptide level ≥300 pg per mL (300 ng per L) Bradycardia (≤50 beats per minute) Rectal examination shows fecal occult blood Anemia (hemoglobin level <9.0 per dL [90.0 g per L]) Chest pain associated with syncope ECG with Q wave (not in lead III) Oxygen saturation ≤94% on room air	Age >65 y History of cardiovascular disease Syncope without a prodrome Abnormal ECG findings	Palpitations preceding syncope Heart disease or abnormal EKG or both Syncope during effort Syncope while supine Precipitating or predisposing factors or both (warm-crowded place, prolonged orthostasis, fear, pain, emotion) Autonomic prodrome (nausea/vomiting)
Accuracy	98% sensitive 56% specific	87% sensitive 66% specific	97% sensitive 73% specific	92% sensitive 69% specific

predicted risk, with one study demonstrating a 30% admission rate for low-risk patients. A review of the American College of Emergency Physicians clinical policy on syncope found that overall admission rates could be cut in half, without missing any high-risk patients, by following the published recommendations.[28] Although a physician's clinical judgement should always take precedence, using algorithms, such as the one suggested by McDermott and Quinn,[29] (**Fig. 1**) will aid in risk stratifying patients presenting with syncope, limit unnecessary testing and

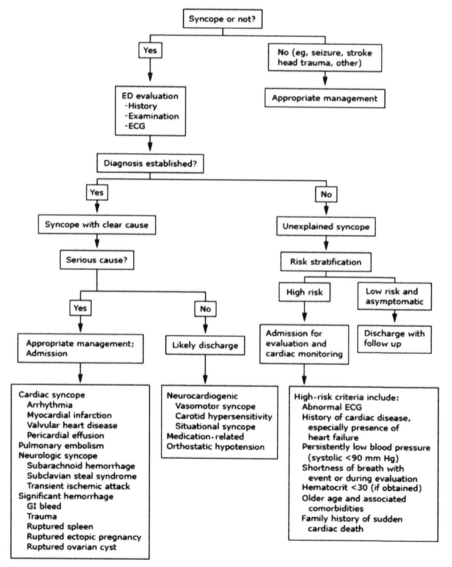

Fig. 1. Algorithm representing the emergency department approach to an adult patient with syncope. ED, emergency department; GI, gastrointestinal. (Reproduced with permission from: McDermott D, Quinn J. Approach to the adult patient with syncope in the emergency department. In: UpToDate, Post TW (Ed), UpToDate, Waltham, MA. (Accessed on 5/27/2016.) Copyright © 2015 UpToDate, Inc. For more information visit www.uptodate.com.)

admissions, and provide substantial cost saving to the health care system without putting patients at risk.

SUMMARY

Syncope is a common medical event that leads to a significant cost burden on the US health system. Part of this cost burden stems from inappropriate use of diagnostic testing in the evaluation of syncope, as well as unnecessary inpatient hospitalizations for syncope. The most cost-effective tools in diagnosing syncope remain a thorough history and physical examination, including the documentation of orthostatic vital signs. All syncope patients should have a resting ECG but routine blood tests, neuro-imaging, echocardiography, and inpatient telemetry monitoring are not routinely warranted because they rarely contribute to the diagnosis but add substantial cost. Although multiple risk stratification tools to identify high-risk patients and diagnostic and management guidelines exist, widespread use of such tools is not commonplace. Therefore, resource utilization in syncope has not been significantly affected by a potential evidence-based, high-value approach.[3] Applying available tools can reduce syncope-related costs substantially without increasing risks to patients.

REFERENCES

1. Lemonick D. Evaluation of syncope in the emergency department. Am J Clin Med 2010;7(1):11–9.
2. Parry SW. An approach to the evaluation and management of syncope in adults. BMJ 2010;340:c880.
3. Probst M, Kanzaria H, Gbedmah M, et al. National trends in resource utilization associate with ED visits for syncope. Am J Emerg Med 2015;33:998–1001.
4. Rosanio S, Schwarz E, Ware D, et al. Syncope in adults: systematic review and proposal of a diagnostic and therapeutic algorithm. Int J Cardiol 2013;162: 149–57.
5. Benditt D, Adkisson W. Approach to the patient with syncope: venues, presentations, diagnoses. Cardiol Clin 2013;31:9–25.
6. Moya A, Sutton R, Ammirati F, et al. Task force for the diagnosis and management of syncope, European Society of Cardiology (ESC), European Heart Rhythm Association (EHRA), Heart Failure Association (HFA), Heart Rhythm Society (HRS). Guidelines for the diagnosis and management of syncope (version 2009). Eur Heart J 2009;30(21):2361–71.
7. Strickberger SA, Benson DW, Biaggioni I, et al. American Heart Association Councils on clinical cardiology, cardiovascular nursing, cardiovascular disease in the young, and stroke; quality of care and outcomes research interdisciplinary working group; American College of Cardiology Foundation; Heart Rhythm Society. AHA/ACCF scientific statement on the evaluation of syncope. J Am Coll Cardiol 2006;47:473–84.
8. Quinn R. What is the most cost-effective evaluation for a first syncopal episode? The Hospitalist. 2010. Available at: http://www.the-hospitalist.org/article/what-is-the-most-cost-effective-evaluation-for-a-first-syncopal-episode/. Accessed September 8, 2015.
9. Lizner M, Yang EH, Estes NA 3rd, et al. Diagnosing syncope. Part 1: value of history, physical examination, and electrocardiography. Clinical efficacy assessment project of the American College of Physicians. Ann Intern Med 1997;126(12): 989–96.

10. Costantino G, Furlan R. Syncope risk stratification in the emergency department. Cardiol Clin 2013;31:27–38.
11. Reed MJ, Newby DE, Coull AJ, et al. The ROSE (risk stratification of syncope in the emergency department) study. J Am Coll Cardiol 2010;55(8):713–21.
12. Sarasin FP, Junod AF, Carballo D, et al. Role of echocardiography in the evaluation of syncope: a prospective study. Heart 2002;88(4):363–7.
13. Kadian-Dodov D, Papolos A, Olin JW. Diagnostic utility of carotid artery duplex ultrasonography in the evaluation of syncope: a good test ordered for the wrong reason. Eur Heart J Cardiovasc Imaging 2015;16(6):621–5.
14. Schnipper JL, Ackerman RH, Krier BA, et al. Diagnostic yield and utility of neurovascular ultrasonography in the evaluation of patients with syncope. Mayo Clin Proc 2005;80(4):480–8.
15. Sarasin FP, Carball D, Slama S, et al. Usefulness of 24-h Holter monitoring in patients with unexplained syncope and a high likelihood of arrhythmias. Int J Cardiol 2005;101:203–7.
16. Rockx MA, Hoch JS, Klein GJ, et al. Is ambulatory monitoring for 'community-acquired' syncope economically attractive? A cost-effectiveness analysis of a randomized trial of external loop recorders versus Holter monitoring. Am Heart J 2005;150:1065.
17. Sivakumaran S, Krahn AD, Klein GJ, et al. A prospective randomized comparison of loop recorders versus Holter monitors in patient with syncope or presyncope. Am J Med 2003;115:1–5.
18. Schuchert A, Mass R, Kretzschmar C, et al. Diagnostic yield of electrocardiographic loop recorders in patients with recurrent syncope and negative tilt table test. Pacing Clin Electrophysiol 2003;26:1837–40.
19. Cooper PN, Westby M, Pitcher DW, et al. Synopsis of the national institute for health and clinical excellence guideline for management of transient loss of consciousness. Ann Intern Med 2011;155:543–9.
20. Krahn AD, Klein GJ, Yee R, et al. Randomized assessment of syncope trial: conventional diagnostic testing versus a prolonged monitoring strategy. Circulation 2001;104:46–51.
21. Brignole M, Ungar A, Bartoletti A, et al. Evaluation of guidelines in syncope study 2 (EGSYS-2) group. Standardized-care pathway vs usual management of syncope patients presenting as emergencies at general hospitals. Europace 2006; 8:644–50.
22. Edvardsson N, Frykman V, van Mechelen R, et al. Use of implantable loop recorders to increase the diagnostic yield in unexplained syncope: results from the PICTURE registry. Europace 2011;13:262–9.
23. Edvardsson N, Wolff C, Tsintzos S, et al. Costs of unstructured investigation of unexplained syncope: insights from a micro-costing analysis of the observational PICTURE registry. Europace 2015;17:1141–8.
24. Sarasin FP, Pruvot E, Louis-Simonet M, et al. Stepwise evaluation of syncope: a prospective population-based controlled study. Int J Cardiol 2008;127:103–11.
25. Grossman SA, Fischer C, Lipsitz LA, et al. Predicting adverse outcomes in syncope. J Emerg Med 2007;33(3):233–9.
26. Quinn JV, Steill IG, McDermott DA, et al. Derivation of the San Francisco Syncope Rule to predict patients with short-term serious outcomes. Ann Emerg Med 2004; 43(2):224–32.
27. Del Rosso A, Ungar A, Maggi R, et al. Clinical predictors of cardiac syncope at initial evaluation in patients referred urgently to general hospital: the EGSYS score. Heart 2008;94:1620–6.

28. Huff JS, Decker WW, Quinn JV, et al. Clinical policy: critical issues in the evaluation and management of adult patients presenting to the emergency department with syncope. Ann Emerg Med 2007;49:431–4.

29. McDermott D, Quinn J. Approach to the adult patient with syncope in the emergency department. From UpToDate. Available at: http://uptodate.com/contents/approach-to-the-adult-patient-with-syncope-in-the-emergency-department. Accessed October 3, 2015.

Evidence-based Evaluation and Management of Chronic Cough

Andreas Achilleos, MD

KEYWORDS

- Chronic cough • Upper airway cough syndrome • Cough variant asthma
- Reflux disease • Nonasthmatic eosinophilic bronchitis
- Cough hypersensitivity syndrome

KEY POINTS

- Chronic cough is a common complaint in the outpatient setting.
- The evaluation of chronic cough is largely based on anatomic diagnostic protocols focused on the most common causes.
- The evidence supporting such protocols is limited and etiologic work-up can occasionally be extensive, costly, and low yield.
- Sequential empiric therapy for the most common causes of chronic cough has thus been recommended instead.
- Focus on the pathophysiologic mechanisms of chronic cough has recently led to the proposal that cough hypersensitivity syndrome is central in its pathogenesis.

INTRODUCTION

The cough reflex is a defense mechanism protecting the lungs from aspiration and also facilitating clearance of secretions, noxious substances, and foreign bodies from the airways.

Cough of any duration is the most common presenting symptom in the primary care setting. According to the National Ambulatory Medical Care Survey from 2010,[1] cough was the primary reason for an outpatient visit in more than 2% of cases. Cough negatively affects patients' quality of life[2–4] and may also lead to severe complications, such as syncope, urine incontinence, rib fractures, pneumothorax, and lung herniation.

Acute cough, which is most commonly caused by a viral upper respiratory illness, typically resolves within 3 weeks. A recent systematic review found that the mean duration of acute cough reported in the literature was about 18 days, contrary to patients' expectation, which was 7 to 9 days.[5]

Internal Medicine Residency Program, Internal Medicine, Hershey Medical Center, 35 Hope Drive, Suite 104, Hershey, PA 17033, USA
E-mail address: aachilleos@hmc.psu.edu

Med Clin N Am 100 (2016) 1033–1045
http://dx.doi.org/10.1016/j.mcna.2016.04.008
0025-7125/16/$ – see front matter © 2016 Elsevier Inc. All rights reserved.

Chronic cough lasts more than 8 weeks and it is self-reported by more than 10% of adults in the community.[6] Chronic cough may last for several years; cause significant physical and psychological distress to the patients; and lead to multiple office visits, extensive testing, as well as referrals to specialists such as allergy, otolaryngology, and pulmonology.[7]

CAUSES OF CHRONIC COUGH

The most common causes of chronic cough include smoking and its long-term consequences, such as chronic obstructive pulmonary disease, angiotensin-converting enzyme (ACE) inhibitor use, upper airway cough syndrome (UACS), airway bronchospasm (asthma) and gastroesophageal reflux disease (GERD).

Angiotensin-converting Enzyme Inhibitors

ACE inhibitors may cause cough in 5% to 20% of patients who receive these medications.[8] This adverse effect is not dose dependent, and may occur anytime during the course of treatment, typically a few days to several months after treatment is initiated. The mechanism behind ACE inhibitor–induced cough is thought to be the accumulation of bradykinin and other substances, which are metabolized by the ACE. ACE inhibitor–induced cough typically resolves within 1 to 4 weeks after discontinuing the ACE inhibitor.[9] Angiotensin receptor blockers (ARBs) are less likely to cause cough compared with ACE inhibitors (rates seem to be similar to placebo) and may be used as an alternative when this side effect warrants discontinuation of the ACE inhibitor. In patients who are nonsmokers, not on treatment with an ACE inhibitor, and have normal chest radiographs, chronic cough is caused by UACS (most common), asthma (second most common), or GERD (third most common) in a large percentage of cases, which may exceed 90%.[10] These conditions may coexist in the same patient and are frequently asymptomatic (silent) besides cough.

Upper Airway Cough Syndrome

UACS (also referred to as postnasal drip or rhinitis) can be caused by allergic rhinitis (seasonal or perennial), nonallergic rhinitis (vasomotor and nonallergic rhinitis with eosinophilia), rhinitis medicamentosa (rebound symptoms after prolonged use of decongestants), infection (chronic bacterial sinusitis), allergic fungal sinusitis, and anatomic abnormalities such as deviated septum. It is not known why some patients with chronic rhinitis or sinusitis go on to develop persistent cough and some do not. UACS can be silent (no symptoms besides cough) in up to 20% of cases.[11] Because of its chronicity it is likely that, over time, patients will become tolerant to other symptoms, which are not as bothersome as cough. The diagnosis of silent UACS can reliably be made only after patients show improvement with prescribed treatment, because there are no pathognomonic features on history, physical examination, and laboratory testing. Questions have thus been raised as to whether silent UACS is a separate entity or should instead be classified as chronic unexplained cough,[12] or even a form of cough hypersensitivity syndrome.

Asthma

Asthma is characterized by airway hyperresponsiveness, variable and reversible airway obstruction, and eosinophilic inflammation of the airways. As in patients with UACS, cough may be the only manifestation of the underlying disease process (cough variant asthma), and other symptoms commonly associated with asthma, such as wheezing, shortness of breath, and chest tightness, may be absent. Unlike silent UACS, the diagnosis of cough variant asthma can be confirmed with laboratory testing (spirometry with or without methacholine challenge). Nonasthmatic eosinophilic bronchitis (NAEB) shares eosinophilic airway inflammation with asthma, but there is no demonstrable airflow limitation or hypersensitivity on spirometry and methacholine testing.[13] The reported frequency of NAEB as a cause of chronic cough varies in different reports. Misclassification is possible because sputum examination or bronchoalveolar lavage to detect airway eosinophilia are not always performed during the diagnostic work-up, and NAEB tends to respond to corticosteroids in the same way as asthma.

Gastroesophageal Reflux Disease

This term encompasses distal esophageal acid exposure, proximal (laryngopharyngeal) exposure to esophageal content with aspiration into the airways, as well as nonacid (or weakly acidic) reflux.[14] Direct effects of gastric acid or esophageal contents on the airways and vagal nerve stimulation from reflux are considered the primary mechanisms for triggering the cough reflex. Other symptoms of acid reflux, such as heartburn, may be scarce or absent (silent reflux) in as many as 75% of cases of reflux-induced cough.[15] Similar to cough variant asthma, laboratory testing (such as impedance-pH esophageal monitoring) may confirm the presence of silent reflux, although, as discussed later in this article, treatment directed at that does not always resolve the cough. More than 1 of the causes discussed earlier may be present in some cases, and up to 40% of patients receive no specific diagnosis after work-up is completed (idiopathic or unexplained cough).[16,17]

Cough Hypersensitivity Syndrome

Cough hypersensitivity syndrome has increasingly been proposed as the underlying mechanism and final common pathway for many of the traditional causes of chronic cough.[18,19] It was recently defined as "troublesome coughing triggered by low level of thermal, mechanical or chemical exposure".[18] It is characterized by enhancement of the cough reflex through sensitization of afferent neuronal pathways of cough, both at the peripheral and central levels. Patients with cough hypersensitivity syndrome develop cough in response to stimuli and their concentrations, which would not otherwise elicit cough. It is thought that this nerve hypersensitivity is a result of various triggers (insults), such as upper respiratory infections and allergic rhinitis. Chronic cough seen with UACS, asthma, and reflux may be perpetuated by the development of cough hypersensitivity. Pharyngeal and/or laryngeal sensations (irritation, tickle, tightness, throat clearing, globus), which are frequently associated with UACS and reflux-induced cough, may represent sensory neuronal dysfunction of vagal afferents in the upper airways and a phenotype of cough hypersensitivity syndrome.[20,21] Symptoms such as dysphonia, dysphagia, dyspnea, and abnormalities of vocal fold motion on laryngoscopy may also be present along with cough as part of the pharyngeal/laryngeal nerve dysfunction seen with cough hypersensitivity syndrome.[22,23] The frequency of cough hypersensitivity syndrome in patients with chronic cough is not known because diagnostic criteria are not established yet, but this diagnosis may apply to many patients diagnosed with idiopathic chronic cough.

Apart from the common causes discussed earlier, many other disorders can cause chronic cough, including chronic lung disease, chronic or indolent respiratory infection such as pertussis, sleep apnea, congestive heart failure, otolaryngology conditions, mediastinal problems and anatomic variants (**Box 1**).

Box 1
Other causes of chronic cough

Chronic lung disease (bronchiectasis, cystic fibrosis, interstitial lung disease, sarcoidosis, bronchiolitis, recurrent aspiration, bronchogenic carcinoma, foreign body, arteriovenous malformations)

Chronic/indolent respiratory infections (pertussis, lung abscess, tuberculosis, fungal, parasitic)

Ear, nose, throat (ENT) problems (vocal cord dysfunction, enlarged tonsils, ear canal cerumen, or foreign body)

Obstructive sleep apnea, congestive heart failure

Psychogenic or habitual cough

Mediastinal problems (retrosternal goiter, aneurysms, aberrant blood vessels such as the innominate or subclavian arteries, fibrosing mediastinitis)

Zenker diverticulum

EVALUATION OF PATIENTS WITH CHRONIC COUGH
History and Physical Examination

Patients should be asked about their smoking status, medications, exposure to allergens or irritants, geographic and occupational factors, as well as other respiratory and systemic symptoms such as fever, chills, anorexia, weight loss, night sweats, hemoptysis, shortness of breath, or chest pain. The presence of any of these symptoms should prompt more urgency in the patient's evaluation, particularly focused on assessing serious conditions such as infections, malignancy, or heart failure.

With regard to UACS, health care providers should obtain a history of environmental allergies, and elicit symptoms of rhinitis (congestion, sneezing, rhinorrhea). As discussed previously, symptoms such as a sensation of foreign body in throat and throat clearing, thought to be specific for UACS, may represent sensitization of the cough reflex, seen with a variety of causes. On physical examination, nasopharyngeal or oropharyngeal secretions, cobblestone appearance of the oropharynx, and presence of nasal polyps may suggest the presence of UACS.

When considering the possibility of asthma, patients with chronic cough should be asked about other symptoms suggestive of that diagnosis, such as wheezing, shortness of breath, and chest tightness. Asthma-related cough may be precipitated by exercise, by allergens such as pollen and animal dander, or by other irritants or cold air. Symptoms of asthma may be worse or even exclusively present at night. A personal or family history of atopic disease should also be elicited. Physical examination may reveal wheezing, especially with forced expiration, as when using a peak flow meter.

For the diagnosis of reflux disease, patients should be asked about symptoms suggestive of acid reflux, such as heartburn, dyspepsia, sour taste, hoarseness, globus sensation, and dysphagia.

As discussed previously, patients with cough hypersensitivity syndrome may have other symptoms suggestive of pharyngeal and laryngeal hypersensitivity, such as throat tickling, irritation or blockage, and dysphonia.

Pertussis outbreaks have increased over the past decade, with more than 48,000 cases reported in the United States in 2012, according to data from the US Centers for Disease Control and Prevention.[24] If pertussis is suspected based on community outbreaks or patient exposure, the history should focus on the presence of inspiratory sounds, paroxysms of cough, post-tussive emesis, and review of the patient's immunization status.

Patients should be asked whether cough is provoked by eating or drinking and whether other symptoms suggestive of aspiration (such as dysphagia, choking) are present.

Sleep apnea has recently been suggested as a cause of chronic cough and physicians should ask for relevant symptoms, such as snoring, daytime somnolence, fatigue, morning headaches. Cough may be primarily nocturnal, whereas acid reflux symptoms may also be present in patients with sleep apnea.[25]

Cough is sometimes the presenting symptom of heart failure; relevant symptoms and signs, such as orthopnea, dyspnea on exertion, and lower extremity edema, should be sought.

With regard to chronic lung disease, physicians should perform a careful examination to detect any adventitious lung sounds such as rales, prolonged expiration, wheezing, finger clubbing, or lymphadenopathy.

A careful ear, nose, and throat examination may detect other potential causes of chronic cough, such as cerumen impaction, boggy nasal turbinates, and enlarged tonsils.

In general, the character of cough (dry or productive) is not thought to be important in the causal diagnosis of chronic cough, although it has been suggested that a significant amount of sputum production is more likely to be associated with primary lung disease such as bronchiectasis or chronic bronchitis.[26]

Diagnostic Testing

When the history, physical examination, and chest radiograph fail to identify a plausible cause of chronic cough, empirical therapeutic trials for common causes of chronic cough such as UACS, asthma, and reflux may be more cost-effective than an exhaustive diagnostic work-up.[27] When undertaken, diagnostic testing for chronic cough is traditionally focused on the most common causes of chronic cough but may also be supplemented at various stages by empirical therapeutic trials, based on the individual patient characteristics and preferences. Physicians should carefully consider the limitations of diagnostic testing for chronic cough, including the occasionally low sensitivity and specificity, invasive character, and cost. Identifying a potential cause of cough during the diagnostic work-up does not always guarantee a response to prescribed treatment. Furthermore, a combination of causes may be present in some patients with chronic cough, so identification of one plausible cause does not preclude the presence of another.

Chest Radiograph

A chest radiograph should be obtained in most patients with chronic cough, smokers or not. One exception may be the identification of a clear precipitating factor, such as the recent prescription of an ACE inhibitor, and documented resolution of cough after addressing that factor. Note that chest radiograph has limited sensitivity for certain chest disorders. For example, up to 10% of patients with interstitial lung diseases may have normal chest radiographs.[28,29] Mediastinal disorders may also go undiagnosed without a computed tomography (CT) scan of the chest.[30]

Computed Tomography Scan of the Chest

A noncontrast CT scan of the chest should be considered for smokers and other patients with chronic cough, when chronic lung disease is suspected based on history, physical examination, and chest radiograph. This scan would be a full-dose diagnostic study, as opposed to the low-dose CT chest used for lung cancer screening.

Computed Tomography Scan of the Sinuses

The diagnosis of UACS is supported by the history and physical examination, and confirmed by cough improvement or resolution after treatment. There is currently no reliable diagnostic test that can establish the diagnosis of UACS. If UACS is strongly suspected and patients respond partially or not at all to empiric treatment, imaging with CT scan of the sinuses may be considered to evaluate for chronic sinusitis, although clinical evidence for this recommendation is lacking.

Pulmonary Function Testing

Pulmonary function testing should be performed in patients suspected of asthma-induced chronic cough. This testing should include spirometry and, if needed, inhaled methacholine challenge. A decrease of less than 20% in forced expiratory volume in 1 second after maximum methacholine challenge has a high negative predictive value for asthma,[31] although prior use of asthma controller medications may reduce the test's sensitivity.[32] In addition to asthma, pulmonary function testing may also aid in the diagnosis of other chronic airway disorders. For example, a low diffusion capacity of carbon monoxide in the lung may support the diagnosis of interstitial lung disease. If there is suspicion for vocal cord dysfunction, such as in patients with dysphonia or stridor, a flow-volume loop should be requested. Costs of common tests used in the evaluation of chronic cough are listed in **Table 1**.

Sputum Examination

Sputum examination may reveal rare infectious causes of chronic cough and also show eosinophilia (>3% eosinophils), such as in asthma and NAEB. Sputum testing may not be easy to perform in patients with dry cough, because sputum may need to be induced with the patient inhaling increasing concentrations of hypertonic saline. The sensitivity of sputum eosinophilia for the diagnosis of asthma varies widely in different studies,[33,34] whereas it is by definition required for the diagnosis of NAEB. An increased exhaled nitric oxide level supports the diagnoses of cough variant asthma and NAEB[35,36] and can be used as an alternative to sputum testing for eosinophilia. Increased exhaled nitric oxide seems to have good correlation with eosinophilic airway inflammation and tends to predict good response to corticosteroid therapy.[37] In summary, sputum examination for eosinophilia or exhaled nitric oxide level may be used for the diagnosis of NAEB after asthma has been excluded, especially if oral corticosteroid therapy is considered.

Testing for GERD

Testing for reflux disease is particularly controversial, because it may be invasive and costly. Establishing a direct causal relationship between the presence of reflux and cough may prove elusive, even after extensive testing. Laryngoscopy to look for

Table 1
Costs of common tests used in the evaluation of chronic cough

	Health Care Blue Book Fair Price ($)	Medicare Physician's Fee Schedule 2015 ($)
Chest radiograph	52	28
CT chest without contrast	326	181
Spirometry	69	36 (spirometry) to 168 (full pulmonary function test)

evidence of laryngopharyngeal reflux and esophageal endoscopy to detect reflux esophagitis may be normal in the presence of reflux and, even when abnormal, findings may be nonspecific. Twenty-four-hour esophageal pH monitoring has traditionally been considered the gold standard for the diagnosis of acid reflux and may in addition establish a direct relationship between episodes of esophageal acidity (pH<4) and cough. pH monitoring may have limited sensitivity in certain situations; for example, when reflux is nonacid (or weakly acid). Barium esophagogram and impedance-pH esophageal monitoring[38] may be used to detect nonacid (or weakly acid) reflux, a form of reflux for which proton pump inhibitor (PPI) treatment is ineffective. Even when these elaborate tests are used for the diagnosis of reflux disease, antireflux treatment is not always successful. It is thus reasonable to try empiric therapy for acid reflux before testing, especially in patients with a suspicion of reflux based on history and physical examination.

Other tests, outlined in **Box 2**, should be used selectively, when there is high suspicion for the relevant disorder.

TREATMENT OF CHRONIC COUGH
Smoking

In patients who are current smokers, smoking cessation should be strongly encouraged. Cough should be expected to resolve within a few weeks of smoking cessation. No further testing is necessary, unless chronic lung disease or another cause of cough is suspected based on history, physical examination, and chest radiograph. Patients and physicians should be alert to changes in the pattern of chronic cough in smokers, something that may indicate a serious disorder. For current or former smokers who meet the United States Preventive Services Task Force screening criteria for lung cancer screening,[41] a thorough discussion of the potential benefits and risks of screening with low-dose CT chest should take place.

Angiotensin-converting Enzyme Inhibitors

In patients on treatment with an ACE inhibitor, when history and physical examination is not suggestive of another cause of chronic cough, discontinuation of the medication for a few weeks should be considered, before any further evaluation. Patients with congestive heart failure treated with an ACE inhibitor may develop cough as a result of their underlying conditions and this should be differentiated from a medication side effect. Cough typically resolves within 1 to 4 weeks of discontinuation of the

---

Box 2
Miscellaneous tests for the evaluation of chronic cough

Allergy testing, especially in cases in which perennial allergic rhinitis is suspected (indoor allergens such as animal dander, dust mites, and mold most commonly implicated).

Pro–brain natriuretic peptide levels and echocardiogram for congestive heart failure.

Polysomnography for sleep apnea.

Testing for bordetella pertussis via nasopharyngeal culture, polymerase chain reaction, or serology.

Tuberculin skin testing (TST) or interferon-gamma release assay for tuberculosis.

Laryngoscopy for vocal cord dysfunction/paralysis, laryngospasm.

Bronchoscopy when lung infection, sarcoidosis, endobronchial tumor, or foreign body is suspected. On rare occasions, bronchoscopy may uncover lesions even when CT chest is unremarkable.[39,40]

ACE inhibitor, but on occasion cough may resolve even while treatment continues. It is thus important in the decision making to weigh any potential adverse effects from discontinuing the medication. ARBs do not generally cause cough and have proven efficacy for most of the conditions in which ACE inhibitor therapy is indicated, such as congestive heart failure, hypertension, and diabetes mellitus with microalbuminuria. In contrast, ACE inhibitors are generally cheaper and have a longer body of evidence supporting their use.[42] If clinically necessary rechallenge with an ACE inhibitor may be attempted, because cough may not recur in some patients.[9]

Nonsmokers, Not on Angiotensin-converting Enzyme Inhibitors and with Normal Chest Radiographs

In patients with chronic cough who are nonsmokers, have normal chest radiographs, and are not receiving an ACE inhibitor, sequential empiric therapy based on initial clinical findings and targeting the 3 most common causes of chronic cough has been proposed as an alternative to extensive diagnostic work-up.[43] If the initial clinical findings are unrevealing, UACS, asthma, and reflux disease can be treated sequentially and in that order. Empiric therapy may be supplemented in various stages by a targeted diagnostic work-up based on the individual patient characteristics and preference. Success rates of empiric therapy are reported to be high[44] and may be cost-effective as well. When implemented, empiric therapy should be appropriately prolonged, which frequently means several weeks, especially for reflux-induced cough, for which treatment with a PPI is recommended for at least 8 weeks. Partial response to any administered therapy may indicate inadequate dose or duration of treatment, as well as the presence of an alternative or multiple causes.

Upper Airway Cough Syndrome

A combination of a first-generation antihistamine and a decongestant has been traditionally proposed for the treatment of UACS.[11] New-generation antihistamines and nasal corticosteroids may be used as an alternative therapy, especially if the underlying cause of UACS is thought to be allergic rhinitis. Treatment duration should be at least 1 week and may be extended to 4 weeks if needed.

Asthma

An inhaled bronchodilator such as a beta-agonist, with or without an inhaled corticosteroid, can be used for empiric therapy for asthma. Before prescribing a bronchodilator, and especially an inhaled corticosteroid, it is prudent to obtain pulmonary function testing and, if needed, methacholine challenge, to establish the diagnosis of asthma. Oral steroids can be used when the suspicion for asthma remains high and in patients who have none or partial response to inhaled corticosteroids or cannot tolerate them. Oral steroids may show an effect sooner than inhaled corticosteroids, which may take several weeks for their full effect to manifest. NAEB does not typically respond to bronchodilators but does respond to corticosteroids (inhaled or oral). Corticosteroids can be prescribed empirically for patients with chronic cough and normal pulmonary function tests with methacholine challenge. The evidence on the effectiveness of inhaled corticosteroids in subacute and chronic cough, when patients with asthma are excluded, is of low quality and inconsistent.[45] If during the work up of chronic cough, asthma has been ruled out and NAEB still remains a possibility, patients may be further tested with sputum examination for eosinophils and exhaled or nasal nitric oxide levels. Alternatively a course of oral corticosteroids can be prescribed empirically to such patients.

Gastroesophageal Reflux Disease

Empiric therapy for reflux-induced cough with a PPI should be prescribed for at least 8 weeks. The clinical evidence on the effectiveness of PPIs for patients with chronic cough and GERD seems to be limited and inconsistent, even when patients are carefully screened for GERD before enrollment.[46,47] Therapies other than PPIs, such as prokinetic agents and H_2 antihistamines, have not been studied adequately for the treatment of extraesophageal manifestations of reflux such as cough. For patients with inadequate response to an appropriate PPI trial, baclofen can be tried, because it may reduce episodes of reflux and has also been studied for the treatment of refractory cough.[48] Antireflux surgery can also be considered as a last resort and after careful deliberation in patients with refractory, reflux-induced cough.[49,50]

Box 3
Stepwise approach to the evaluation and management of chronic cough

Step 1

Focused treatment based on history and physical examination

Chest radiograph, smoking cessation

Discontinue/substitute ACE inhibitor

Step 2

Consider CT scan of the chest for:
1. Smokers who meet criteria for lung cancer screening
2. Abnormal chest radiograph
3. Presence of red flag symptoms, such as anorexia, weight loss, hemoptysis, fever, or chills
4. Clinical findings of chronic lung disease, such as bibasilar rales, shortness of breath, clubbing

Step 3

Empiric treatment of UACS with antihistamine/decongestant or nasal corticosteroid

Step 4

Spirometry ± bronchoprovocation with methacholine

If positive for asthma, treat with bronchodilators ± inhaled corticosteroids

If negative for asthma, test for NAEB with sputum examination for eosinophilia, exhaled or nasal nitric oxide levels or treat empirically with a course of oral corticosteroids

Consider exhaled nitric oxide testing or sputum testing for eosinophilia before steroid use

Step 5

High-dose PPI and lifestyle changes to address acid reflux, for 8 to 12 weeks

Step 6

Neuromodulator trial for cough hypersensitivity syndrome

Step 7

CT scan of the chest if not already done

Speech therapy evaluation and treatment

Step 8

Consider ENT evaluation for laryngoscopy

Consider gastroenterology evaluation for esophageal impedance-pH monitoring

Consider pulmonology evaluation for bronchoscopy

Cough Hypersensitivity Syndrome

Diagnostic criteria have not been established for cough hypersensitivity syndrome but empiric therapy directed at this syndrome should be considered, especially if therapeutic trials for UACS, asthma, NAEB, and reflux disease have been tried without success. Centrally acting neuromodulators such as amitriptyline, gabapentin, and pregabalin have been shown to improve cough and quality of life in patients with refractory cough.[51–54] The effectiveness of these neuromodulators supports the increasingly prominent hypothesis of cough hypersensitivity syndrome in the pathogenesis of chronic cough. Medications that block receptors on the vagal afferent nerves are currently under investigation.[55]

In patients with cough refractory to the above interventions, speech therapy may be of value, used with[52] or without a neuromodulator.[56] Speech therapy consists of patient education, and respiratory and laryngeal muscle exercises to afford better control of the urge to cough. It may also address voice disorders such as dysphonia and hoarseness, which may accompany chronic cough.

Symptomatic treatment with cough suppressants such as dextromethorphan, codeine, and benzonatate; expectorants; or mucolytics may also be considered, although the evidence on the effectiveness of such medications is insufficient[57,58] and their use may be compounded by side effects.

It is also important to offer patient reassurance, because the cause of chronic cough is usually benign, as well as education regarding the expected duration of symptoms. When seeking evaluation for chronic cough, patients may be more concerned about the underlying cause than about the symptom.[59] Identifying the specific patient concern allows individualization of the extent of the diagnostic evaluation and treatment (**Box 3**).

SUMMARY/FUTURE CONSIDERATIONS

Most patients with chronic cough respond to empiric therapy that is based on the initial clinical evaluation and directed toward the most common causes, as outlined earlier. Such therapy should in most cases precede extensive etiologic work-up, because testing can be invasive, costly, and low yield.

The evidence supporting current recommendations for diagnosis and treatment of chronic cough has significant limitations[60] and further research is needed. Specifically, more research is needed to establish the comparative effectiveness, including long-term outcomes, and cost-effectiveness of empiric therapy versus more extensive diagnostic testing, especially in view of the availability of novel treatments (nasal corticosteroids for UACS, neuromodulators for cough hypersensitivity syndrome, speech therapy) and tests such as exhaled nitric oxide for the diagnosis of some of the most common causes of chronic cough.

The ability to diagnose UACS and reflux-induced cough, while at the same time predicting who will respond to available treatments, remains limited. The pathophysiology and some of the symptoms associated with these diagnoses may overlap with the cough hypersensitivity syndrome.

Further information is needed to allow clinicians to better clarify and define the abnormalities of the cough reflex that constitute the cough hypersensitivity syndrome, the role of neuromodulator therapy in the treatment of chronic cough, and how best to integrate these into the current paradigm for the evaluation and management of chronic cough.

REFERENCES

1. Available at: http://www.cdc.gov/nchs/data/ahcd/nhamcs_outpatient/2010_opd_web_tables.pdf.
2. Chamberlain S, Garrod R, Douiri A, et al. The impact of chronic cough: a cross-sectional European survey. Lung 2015;193:401–8.
3. Young EC, Smith JA. Quality of life in patients with chronic cough. Ther Adv Respir Dis 2010;4(1):49–55.
4. Polley L, Yaman N, Heaney L, et al. Impact of cough across different chronic respiratory diseases: comparison of two cough-specific health-related quality of life questionnaires. Chest 2008;134(2):295–302.
5. Ebell M, Lundgren J, Youngpairoj S. How long does a cough last? Comparing patients' expectations with data from a systematic review of the literature. Ann Fam Med 2013;11(1):5–13.
6. Ford AC, Forman D, Moayyedi P, et al. Cough in the community: a cross sectional survey and the relationship to gastrointestinal symptoms. Thorax 2006;61:975–9.
7. Song WJ, Chang YS, Faruqi S, et al. The global epidemiology of chronic cough in adults: a systematic review and meta-analysis. Eur Respir J 2015;45(5):1479–81.
8. Israili ZH, Hall WD. Cough and angioneurotic edema associated with angiotensin-converting enzyme inhibitor therapy. A review of the literature and pathophysiology. Ann Intern Med 1992;117:234–42.
9. Dicpinigaitis PV. Angiotensin-converting enzyme inhibitor-induced cough: ACCP evidence-based clinical practice guidelines. Chest 2006;129(Suppl 1):169S–73S.
10. Pratter MR. Overview of common causes of chronic cough. ACCP evidence-based clinical practice guidelines. Chest 2006;129:59S–62S.
11. Pratter MR. Chronic upper airway cough syndrome secondary to rhinosinus diseases (previously referred to as postnasal drip syndrome). ACCP evidence-based clinical practice guidelines. Chest 2006;129:63S–71S.
12. Birring SS. Controversies in the evaluation and management of chronic cough. Am J Respir Crit Care Med 2011;183(6):708–15.
13. Brightling CE. Chronic cough due to nonasthmatic eosinophilic bronchitis. ACCP evidence-based clinical practice guidelines. Chest 2006;129:116S–21S.
14. Patterson N, Mainie I, Rafferty G, et al. Nonacid reflux episodes reaching the pharynx are important factors associated with cough. J Clin Gastroenterol 2009;43(5):414–9.
15. Irwin RS. Chronic cough due to gastroesophageal reflux disease. ACCP evidence-based clinical practice guidelines. Chest 2006;129:80S–94S.
16. Haque RA, Usmani OS, Barnes PJ. Chronic idiopathic cough: a discrete clinical entity? Chest 2005;127:1710–3.
17. Pratter MR. Unexplained (idiopathic) cough. ACCP evidence-based clinical practice guidelines. Chest 2006;129:220S–1S.
18. Chung KF, Canning B, McGarvey L. Eight International London Cough Symposium 2014: cough hypersensitivity syndrome as the basis for chronic cough. Pulm Pharmacol Ther 2015;35:76–80.
19. Song WJ, Chang YS. Cough hypersensitivity as a neuro-immune interaction. Clin Transl Allergy 2015;5:24.
20. Yu L, Xu X, Lv H, et al. Advances in upper airway cough syndrome. Kaohsiung J Med Sci 2015;31(5):223–8.
21. Hilton E, Marsden P, Thurston A, et al. Clinical features of the urge-to-cough in patients with chronic cough. Respir Med 2015;109(6):701–7.

22. Altman KW, Noordzij JP, Rosen CA, et al. Neurogenic cough. Laryngoscope 2015;125(7):1675–81.

23. Hull JH, Menon A. Laryngeal hypersensitivity in chronic cough. Pulm Pharmacol Ther 2015;35:111–6.

24. Available at: http://www.cdc.gov/pertussis/surv-reporting/cases-by-year.html.

25. Chan K, Ing A, Birring SS. Cough in obstructive sleep apnoea. Pulm Pharmacol Ther 2015;35:129–31.

26. Martin MJ, Harrison TW. Causes of chronic productive cough: An approach to management. Respir Med 2015;109(9):1105–13.

27. Lin L, Poh KL, Lim TK. Empirical treatment of chronic cough–a cost-effectiveness analysis. Proc AMIA Symp 2001;383–7.

28. Brown KK. Chronic cough due to chronic interstitial pulmonary diseases. ACCP evidence-based clinical practice guidelines. Chest 2006;129:180S–5S.

29. Epler GR, McLoud TC, Gaensler EA, et al. Normal chest roentgenograms in chronic diffuse infiltrative lung disease. N Engl J Med 1978;298:934–9.

30. Theofilos D, Triantafillidou C, Zetos A, et al. 44-year-old man with chronic cough, weakness, and a mediastinum mass. Chest 2015;148(3):e86–90.

31. American Thoracic Society. Guidelines for methacholine and exercise challenge testing-1999. Am J Respir Crit Care Med 2000;161:309–29.

32. Sumino K, Sugar EA, Irvin CG, et al. Methacholine challenge test: diagnostic characteristics in asthmatic patients receiving controller medications. J Allergy Clin Immunol 2012;130(1):69–75.

33. Hunter CJ, Brightling CE, Woltmann G, et al. A comparison of the validity of different diagnostic tests in adults with asthma. Chest 2002;121(4):1051–7.

34. Douwes J, Gibson P, Pekkanen J, et al. Non eosinophilic asthma: importance and possible mechanism. Thorax 2002;57:643–8.

35. Maniscalco M, Faraone S, Matteo S, et al. Extended analysis of exhaled and nasal nitric oxide for the evaluation of chronic cough. Respir Med 2015;109: 970–4.

36. Kowal K, Bodzenta-Lukaszyk K, Zukowski S. Exhaled nitric oxide in evaluation of young adults with chronic cough. J Asthma 2009;46:692–8.

37. Dweik R, Boggs P, Erzurum S, et al. An official ATS clinical practice guideline: interpretation of exhaled nitric oxide levels (Fe_{NO}) for clinical applications. Am J Respir Crit Care Med 2011;184(5):602–15.

38. Ribolsi M, Savarino E, De Bortoli N, et al. Reflux pattern and role of impedance-pH variables in predicting PPI response in patients with suspected GERD-related chronic cough. Aliment Pharmacol Ther 2014;40:966–73.

39. Behnia MM, Catalano PW. A 54-year-old woman with chronic cough and an endobronchial mass. Tanaffos 2011;10(2):72–4.

40. Decalmer S, Woodcock A, Greaves M, et al. Airway abnormalities at flexible bronchoscopy in patients with chronic cough. Eur Respir J 2007;30(6):1138–42.

41. Available at: http://www.uspreventiveservicestaskforce.org/Page/Document/UpdateSummaryFinal/lung-cancer-screening.

42. Li EC, Heran BS, Wright JM. Angiotensin converting enzyme (ACE) inhibitors versus angiotensin receptor blockers for primary hypertension. Cochrane Database Syst Rev 2014;(8):CD009096.

43. Pratter MR, Brightling CE, Boulet LP, et al. An empiric integrative approach to the management of cough. ACCP evidence-based clinical practice guidelines. Chest 2006;129:222S–31S.

44. Deng HY, Luo W, Zhang M, et al. Initial empirical treatment based on clinical feature of chronic cough. Clin Respir J 2015. http://dx.doi.org/10.1111/crj.1227.

45. Johnstone KJ, Chang AB, Fong KM, et al. Inhaled corticosteroids for subacute and chronic cough in adults. Cochrane Database Syst Rev 2013;(3):CD009305.

46. Chang AB, Lasserson TJ, Gaffney J, et al. Gastro-oesophageal reflux treatment for prolonged non-specific cough in children and adults. Cochrane Database Syst Rev 2011;(1):CD004823.

47. Kahrilas PJ, Howden CW, Hughes N, et al. Response of chronic cough to acid-suppressive therapy in patients with gastroesophageal reflux disease. Chest 2013;143(3):605–12.

48. Han-Jing LV, Qiu ZM. Refractory chronic cough due to gastroesophageal reflux: Definition, mechanism and management. World J Methodol 2015;5(3):149–56.

49. Hoppo T, Komatsu Y, Jobe BA. Antireflux surgery in patients with chronic cough and abnormal proximal exposure as measured by hypopharyngeal multichannel intraluminal impedance. JAMA Surg 2013;148(7):608–16.

50. Lugaresi M, Aramini B, Daddi N, et al. Effectiveness of antireflux surgery for the cure of chronic cough associated with gastroesophageal reflux disease. World J Surg 2015;39(1):208–15.

51. Ryan NM, Birring SS, Gibson PG. Gabapentin for refractory chronic cough: a randomised, double-blind, placebo-controlled trial. Lancet 2012;380(9853):1583–9.

52. Vertigan AE, Kapela SL, Ryan NM, et al. Pregabalin and speech pathology combination therapy for refractory chronic cough: a randomised controlled trial. Chest 2016;149(3):639–48.

53. Gibson PG, Vertigan AE. Gabapentin in chronic cough. Pulm Pharmacol Ther 2015;35:145–8.

54. Gibson P, Wang G, McGarvey L, et al. Treatment of unexplained chronic cough: CHEST guideline and expert panel report. Chest 2016;149(1):27–44.

55. Abdulqawi R, Dockry R, Holt K, et al. P2X3 receptor antagonist (AF-219) in refractory chronic cough: a randomised, double-blind, placebo-controlled phase 2 study. Lancet 2015;385:1198–205.

56. Gibson PG, Vertigan AE. Speech pathology for chronic cough: a new approach. Pulm Pharmacol Ther 2009;22(2):159–62.

57. McCrory DC, Coeytaux RR, Yancy WS Jr, et al. Assessment and Management of Chronic Cough. Rockville (MD): Agency for Healthcare Research and Quality (US); 2013.

58. Yancy WS Jr, McCrory DC, Coeytaux RR, et al. Efficacy and tolerability of treatments for chronic cough: a systematic review and meta-analysis. Chest 2013;144(6):1827–38.

59. Pavord ID, Chung KF. Chronic cough 2. Management of chronic cough. Lancet 2008;371:1375–8.

60. French CT, Diekemper RL, Irwin RS. Assessment of intervention fidelity and recommendations for researchers conducting studies on the diagnosis and treatment of chronic cough in the adult: CHEST guideline and expert panel report. Chest 2015;148(1):32–54.

The Approach to Occult Gastrointestinal Bleed

Edgar R. Naut, MD

KEYWORDS

- Occult gastrointestinal bleeding • Obscure gastrointestinal bleeding
- Small bowel bleeding

KEY POINTS

- Occult bleeding is not visible and may present with positive fecal occult blood test or iron deficiency anemia.
- Obscure bleeding can be overt or occult, with no source identified despite diagnostic workup.
- The small bowel has been identified as the cause of obscure gastrointestinal bleeding in most patients.
- Video capsule endoscopy should be considered first for small bowel investigation followed by any form of deep enteroscopy when endoscopic evaluation or therapy is required.

INTRODUCTION

Gastrointestinal (GI) bleeding encompasses all bleeding that occurs in the GI tract, which extends from the mouth to the large bowel.[1] The different types of GI bleeding are classified based on their clinical presentation as overt, obscure, or occult.[2] *Overt GI bleeding* is visible clinically and used to describe hematemesis, hematochezia, or melena.[2] *Obscure GI bleeding* refers to recurrent bleeding for which no source is identified on multiple diagnostic modalities including upper endoscopy, colonoscopy, or small bowel radiography.[2] Obscure GI bleeding can either be classified as overt or occult, based on clinical presentation.[2-6] *Occult GI bleeding* is bleeding that is not visible to the patient or the physician. It is detected by either a positive fecal occult blood test (FOBT), or iron deficiency anemia with or without a positive FOBT.[2,5] Before the introduction of video capsule endoscopy (VCE), the term obscure GI bleeding was used and this could be overt or occult.[3-5] Occult obscure bleeding were classified on the presence of iron deficiency anemia with or without a positive FOBT.[4]

Disclosure: The author has nothing to disclose.
Saint Francis Hospital and Medical Center, 114 Woodland Street, Hartford, CT 06105, USA
E-mail address: enaut@stfranciscare.org

Med Clin N Am 100 (2016) 1047–1056
http://dx.doi.org/10.1016/j.mcna.2016.04.013   **medical.theclinics.com**
0025-7125/16/$ – see front matter © 2016 Elsevier Inc. All rights reserved.

Recent guidelines have proposed an update in the terminology used to describe small intestinal bleeding.[4] The proposed changes suggest that the term *occult small bowel bleeding* be reserved for patients presenting with iron deficiency anemia with or without guaiac-positive stools who are found to have a small bowel source of bleeding.[4] The reason for the suggested change is that, given the advances in small bowel imaging, the majority of these patients (75%) have been found to have a small bowel source.[4]

Given the high incidence and the elusiveness of the diagnosis, occult GI bleeding has been associated with an increase in resource use, including prolonged hospitalizations and procedures.[3] Effectiveness in the treatment of occult GI bleeding can be defined as the ability to diagnose, reduce, or stop GI bleeding. It can also be measured by the impact on overall life expectancy to the individual, or the impact to health-related quality of life.[6] The least costly approach to evaluating occult GI bleeding remains uncertain.[3]

The concept of cost effectiveness in health care was introduced in the 1970s to help physicians determine optimal therapies for their patients.[7,8] The question raised is whether the use of a new technology or medication is favored if it is more cost effective.[6] In this review, the diagnostic modalities available to aid in the diagnosis and treatment of occult intestinal bleeding will be discussed to provide clinicians with an evidence-based and cost-effective approach to care.

ETIOLOGY AND PATHOPHYSIOLOGY

The prevalence of small bowel bleeding is approximately 5% to 10% of patients presenting with GI bleeding.[1,4,9] About 10% to 20% of patients presenting with GI bleeding have an unclear etiology despite a full workup, and are considered to be obscure bleeds.[1,4,5,9] Given that most occult GI bleeding is from the small intestine, we focus on causes of bleeding originating from the small intestine. Small bowel bleeding is defined as bleeding that occurs from the region between the ligament of Treitz and ileocecal valve.[9] Causes of small bowel bleeding can be divided as common or uncommon, further dividing common causes by age. **Table 1** lists common etiologies of small intestinal bleeding.

The most common lesions responsible for small bowel bleeding are vascular, with other causes being benign tumors, inflammatory lesions, and medications.[9] Other rare causes include hemophilia, haemosuccus pancreaticus, and aortoenteric fistula.[9]

- Angiodysplasia (angioextasia or vascular ectasia) are abnormally dilated, tortuous, thin-walled vessels, involving capillaries, veins, and arteries. They are visualized within the mucosal and submucosal layers of the gut. They are lined by endothelium with little or no smooth muscle, and lack inflammatory or fibrotic changes.[9] They are the most common cause of small bowel bleeds, particularly in patients older than 40 years of age.[4,9]
- Telangiectasias are different then angiodysplasias because, in addition to involving the GI tract mucosa, they usually have cutaneous and mucous membrane involvement. They lack capillaries and consist of direct connections between arteries and veins and they have excessive layers of smooth muscle without elastic fibers.[9]
- Dieulafoy's lesion is a rare cause of GI bleeding and is usually located in the stomach but can be located in the small intestine.[9,10] These lesions are purely arterial and do not exhibit similarities with arteriovenous malformations or varicose vessels.[10]

Table 1
Causes of small intestinal bleeding

Common Causes		Rare Causes
Under Age 40 y	**Over Age 40 y**	**Henoch–Schoenlein Purpura**
Inflammatory bowel disease	Angioectasia	Small bowel varices and/or portal
Dieulafoy's lesions	Dieulafoy's lesions	hypertensive enteropathy
Neoplasia	Neoplasia	Amyloidosis
Meckel's diverticulum	NSAID ulcers	Blue rubber bleb nevus syndrome
Polyposis syndromes		Pseudoxanthoma elasticum
		Osler–Weber–Rendu syndrome
		Kaposi's sarcoma with AIDS
		Plummer–Vinson syndrome
		Ehlers–Danlos syndrome
		Inherited polyposis syndromes
		(FAP, Peutz–Jeghers)
		Malignant atrophic papulosis
		Hematobilia
		Aortoenteric fistula
		Hemosuccus entericus

Abbreviations: FAP, familial adenomatous polyposis; NSAID, nonsteroidal antiinflammatory drug.
   From Gerson LB, Fidler JL, Cave DR, et al. ACG clinical guideline: diagnosis and management of small bowel bleeding. Am J Gastroenterol 2015;110(9):1269; with permission.

- Small bowel varices: Are large, portosystemic venous collaterals occurring in the small intestine. They are associated with portal hypertension or abdominal surgery and are a rare cause of GI bleeding.[9]
- Small bowel tumors: Uncommon cause of GI bleeding, with primary small bowel tumors accounting for 5% of all primary GI tract neoplasms.[9]
- GI stromal tumors are believed to originate from the intestinal cells of Cajal with the small intestine being the second most common location (30%–35%).[9]
- Small bowel ulcers are an important etiology for small intestinal bleeding and can be multifactorial including inflammatory bowel disease, medications such as nonsteroidal antiinflammatory drugs, or infections such as tuberculosis.[1,2,9]
- Meckel's diverticulum is a common congenital abnormality of the small bowel. It is the result of incomplete closure of the vitelline duct. The bleeding usually results from the ulceration of the ectopic gastric mucosa within the diverticulum.[9]
- Aortoenteric fistula is a rare, life-threatening condition and almost always secondary to reconstructive aortic aneurysmal surgery.[9]
- Hemobilia is a rare cause of bleeding from the small intestine owing to a communication between the vessels and the biliary system.[4,9]
- Haemosuccus pancreaticus is an unusual cause of GI bleeding from the pancreatic blood vessel into the pancreatic duct. It can occur with acute or chronic pancreatitis.[9]

PATIENT HISTORY

A thorough history is the first step to evaluating a patient with an occult GI bleed. This should be followed by a targeted GI history. A patient with a history of GI bleeding, surgical interventions, or other pathology may give some clues as to the source.[2] Unintentional weight loss may suggest a malignancy. Abdominal pain in a patient taking nonsteroidal antiinflammatory drugs may suggest an ulcer. The use of medications such as anticoagulants or antiplatelet agents may precipitate previously undiagnosed lesions. A history of a bleeding diathesis such as with von Willebrand disease may also be illuminating.[4] Surgical and procedure history such as gastric bypass, liver biopsy, liver transplantation, abdominal aortic aneurysm repair, or small bowel resection may suggest sources of blood loss or malabsorption.[2,4] A history of liver disease may suggest bleeding related to portal hypertension. Other historical elements may lead one to a diagnosis of angiodysplasia. These may include chronic kidney disease, renal replacement therapy, aortic stenosis, hypertension, ischemic heart disease, arrhythmias, valvular heart disease, congestive heart failure, chronic respiratory conditions, prior venous thromboembolism, and anticoagulant use.[9,11] A history of long distance running may also lead to GI bleeding secondary to transient intestinal ischemia from decreased splanchnic perfusion during exercise.[2,12] A family history of GI bleeding may suggest hereditary hemorrhagic telangiectasia.[2] Furthermore, a family history of cancer occurring at an early age, particularly colorectal or endometrial, may suggest the presence of hereditary nonpolyposis colorectal cancer (Lynch syndrome).[1]

One of the most important elements of the patient history is age.[1,2,4,9] Age has been known to be a strong determinate for the type of small bowel pathology detected as noted in **Table 1**.[4] Patients under the age of 40 are more likely to have inflammatory bowel disease, whereas those over the age of 40 more likely suffer from angioectasia or ulcers secondary to nonsteroidal anti-inflammatory drugs.[2,4,9]

PHYSICAL EXAMINATION

As with the patient's history, a focused physical examination may reveal clues as to the source of the blood loss. A detailed dermatologic evaluation may be useful in detecting thrombocytopenia, hereditary hemorrhagic telangiectasia, or blue-rubber bleb nevus syndrome.[1,2,4] Other useful physical examination findings that may suggest underlying systemic conditions include dermatitis herpetiformis (celiac disease), erythema nodosum (inflammatory bowel disease), atrophic tongue and brittle spoon-shaped nails (Plummer-Vinson syndrome), hyperextensible joints and ocular and dental abnormalities (Ehlers-Danlos syndrome), and freckles on the lips and in the mouth (Peutz-Jeghers syndrome).[2] The examination should also look for signs of chronic liver, heart, and respiratory conditions.[9,11]

INITIAL MANAGEMENT OF OCCULT GASTROINTESTINAL BLEEDING

It is not uncommon for iron deficiency to be the cause for a presenting chief complaint or found during evaluation of a patient for anemia. Similarly, a positive FOBT is also encountered on a regular basis, be it during routine testing such as during a hospital visit or as a choice in screening for colorectal cancer. The current recommendations for colorectal cancer screening via FOBT include Hemoccult Sensa, which is an improved guaiac based card for FOBT, fecal immunochemical test (FIT) for blood, or fecal DNA. The FIT test is the preferred test because the overall evidence for the Hemoccult Sensa is less than that supporting FIT. FIT testing is preferred when compared with fecal DNA testing do to the higher cost of fecal DNA testing. In addition, FIT testing has an equal and sometimes superior specificity when compared with fecal DNA testing.[13]

ENDOSCOPY AND OTHER DIAGNOSTIC TESTS
Isolated Iron Deficiency Anemia

Iron deficiency anemia occurs in 2% to 5% of adult men and postmenopausal women in the developed world.[14] Despite the high prevalence, very few published guidelines on investigations and management are available, and with a low quality of evidence.[14] When evaluating patients with iron deficiency anemia who are men or postmenopausal women, it is assumed they have GI blood loss even with a negative FOBT.[1,2,14] In premenopausal women, menses may explain iron deficiency anemia. However, colonic and upper GI tract tumors are also reported in this group. In addition to heavy menses, all patients should be evaluated for extraintestinal causes such as epistaxis and hematuria. If heavy menses cannot explain the iron deficiency in premenopausal women or if GI symptoms are present, it is generally accepted that the patient should be evaluated for GI causes.[2,4,6,14] Evaluation involves a colonoscopy and/or esophagogastroduodenal endoscopy followed by VCE if both are negative. In addition, celiac serology should be considered for all adults with iron deficiency anemia.[15]

The justification for this extensive workup for iron deficiency is that physicians often cease investigation of iron deficiency after a negative esophagogastroduodenal endoscopy and colonoscopy, leaving about 30% of patients without a diagnosis.[14] Chronic iron deficiency anemia is known to be associated with high mortality and morbidity, and accounts for a significantly impaired quality of life, placing a huge burden on health care resources.[6,14,16] Without an accurate diagnosis, treatment is limited to empirical iron replacement and blood transfusions, which is often suboptimal for correction of anemia.[14,16] Current recommendations support upper and lower endoscopies; however, there are no clear guidelines about which procedure should be performed first or if a second procedure is necessary if a source is found on the first study.[15] In patients with a negative colonoscopy and esophagogastroduodenal endoscopy on initial testing, repeat endoscopy should be considered as shown in **Fig. 1**.

The current guidelines suggest that a second look endoscopy may have value, given that some studies have shown the high prevalence of missed bleeding lesions within reach of conventional upper and lower endoscopy. This is particularly true when bleeding is overt and less clear cut for occult–obscure bleeding. The current guidelines suggest that a possible alternative instead of standard endoscopy would be a push endoscopy to examine the distal duodenum and proximal jejunum. In addition, every effort should be made to intubate the terminal ilium to visualize the ileal mucosa and to inspect for blood coming from a more proximal location of the small intestine.[4] However, the guidelines do acknowledge that VCE may be an appropriate next step; some studies have shown that repeat endoscopy may not to be cost effective.[4,5,17]

VCE was introduced for clinical use in the United States in 2001 and there are 3 platforms available for clinical use. VCE measures 26×11 mm,[2] and it can take images at a rate of 2 frames per second over a period of 8 to 12 hours. The images are then transmitted to a recording device, and can be downloaded and viewed with the appropriate software.[4] This allows for the noninvasive evaluation of the entire small bowel in 79% to 90% of patients, with a diagnostic yield of 38% to 83%.[4] VCE has a high positive (94%–97%) and negative predictive values (83%–100%) in the evaluation of the GI tract.[4] The findings on VCE frequently lead to endoscopic or surgical intervention or a change in medical management. In addition, 50% to 66% of patients remained transfusion free after VCE-directed interventions.[4]

The yield of VCE is higher in patients with hemoglobin levels of less than 10 g/dL, longer duration of bleeding, multiple episodes of bleeding, overt versus occult bleeding, and performing the test within 2 weeks of a bleeding episode.[4] Limitations include lack of therapeutic capabilities, inability to control its movement through the GI tract, and lack of specificity.[4,18] The main complication is retention of the capsule, which limits its use in patients believed to be obstructed. Studies have shown VCE to

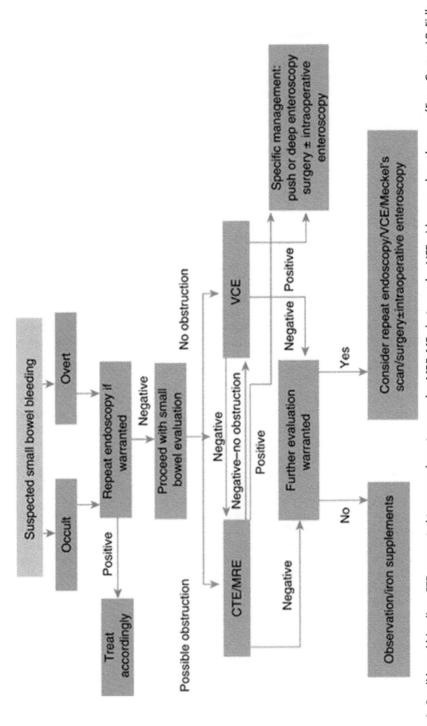

Fig. 1. Small bowel bleeding. CTE, computed tomography enterography; MRE, MR elastography; VCE, video capsule endoscopy. (*From* Gerson LB, Fidler JL, Cave DR, et al. ACG clinical guideline: diagnosis and management of small bowel bleeding. Am J Gastroenterol 2015;110(9):1268; with permission.)

be a cost-effective first step in the evaluation of occult–obscure GI bleeding.[19,20] This is particularly true in centers with limited experience with more advanced endoscopic techniques, such as double balloon endoscopy.[3] A positive VCE would lead to specific management with push or deep enteroscopy with or without intraoperative entero-scopy (IOE). A push enteroscopy is an extended upper endoscopy performed using a long endoscope. Deep enteroscopy or balloon-assisted enteroscopy use the princi-ple of push and pull enteroscopy and finally IOE involves evaluating the small bowel at laparotomy and may be performed orally, rectally or via an enterotomy.

If the VCE is negative, then the patient should be evaluated for further testing versus observation with a trial of iron supplementation. As shown in **Fig. 1**, it is prudent to observe on iron supplements in certain patients who are asymptomatic with negative upper and lower endoscopies and a negative VCE.[2,4] There are no standard recom-mendations for follow-up after initiating iron therapy for iron deficiency; however, a suggested approach is to recheck complete blood counts every 3 months for 1 year and recheck 12 months later if the hemoglobin and red blood cell indices remain normal.[15] An alternative approach is to check the patient periodically with no further follow-up if the blood work is normal and the patient is asymptomatic. There is no role for red blood cell scan, computed tomographic angiography, or angiography in occult GI bleeding; however, these tests are considered diagnostic and therapeutic options in patients with overt GI bleeding.[4]

As noted, several modalities are capable of visualizing the GI tract beyond the scope normal endoscopies. These include balloon-assisted enteroscopy. These can be dou-ble or single balloon enteroscopy. Both types have an overtube with balloons at their distal ends. The double balloon endoscope (DBE) uses a balloon at the end of the scope and in the overtube. The single balloon endoscope uses the tip as an anchor with a single balloon. The DBE can be advanced a distance of 240 to 360 cm distal to the pylorus with the oral approach and the 102 to 140 cm proximal to the ileocecal valve with the rectal approach.[4] DBE has the advantage over VCE in that it is both diagnostic and therapeutic. The diagnostic yield of DBE ranges from 60% to 80% in patients with suspected small bowel bleeding and therapeutic success 40% to 73% of patients.[4] The main limitations of DBE include its invasive nature, prolonged proce-dure time, and requirements for additional personnel. The overall complication rate has been reported to be 1.2%.[4] The theory and technique of single balloon endoscopy are very similar to that DBE.

Spiral Enteroscopy

Spiral enteroscopy consist of a unique overtube with an outer raised spiral ridge at its distal end through which a single balloon endoscope or a DBE can be inserted. It is a 2-person procedure requiring a physician and a nurse. Questions have been raised about some safety concerns with regards to bowel trauma and difficulty in rapid removal in an emergency. However, there have been no major complications reported in the early literature.[4]

Intraoperative Enteroscopy

IOE, the most invasive procedure, involves evaluation of the small bowel at laparot-omy, and may be performed orally, rectally, or via an enterotomy, wherein the scope is inserted through a surgical incision in the small bowel. It is the most reliable method to achieve a complete small bowel evaluation. The procedure has a high mortality rate and should be reserved for refractory bleeding or in patients with a comprehensive negative evaluation or in whom deep enteroscopy cannot be performed because of lysis of adhesions.[4]

DOUBLE BALLOON ENTEROSCOPY VERSUS VIDEO CAPSULE ENDOSCOPY: COST-EFFECTIVENESS ANALYSIS

In 2015, the American College of Gastroenterology provided a cost-effectiveness analysis that compared various diagnostic modalities (push enteroscopy, DBE, VCE-guided DBE, angiography, and IOE), found that DBE was not only the most cost-effective approach in the evaluation of obscure small bowel bleeding, but also had the highest success rate for bleeding cessation.[4,7] However, the investigators concluded that VCE-directed DBE may be associated with better long-term outcomes because of potential for fewer complications and decreased use of endoscopic resources.[7] This is in contrast with another study that concluded that VCE is a cost-saving approach in the evaluation of patients with obscure GI bleeding.[19] A cost analysis study concluded that when looking at workflow management of VCE and DBE from a third-party payer's perspective, a strategy incorporating VCE seems to minimize cost.[21] Other studies have concluded that given the current reimbursement climate for DBE relative to its prolonged procedure time, the fixed cost of capital investment, and the technical skill required to perform the procedure, DBE capacity would likely remain low. It is therefore likely that VCE will be viewed as a viable initial test in the evaluation of occult–obscure GI bleeding.[3]

Positive Fecal Occult Blood Test with or Without Iron Deficiency Anemia

The approach to a positive FOBT test is similar to the approach to isolated iron deficiency (see **Fig. 1**). If a source of bleeding is not found after the performance of a standard upper and lower endoscopic examination, small bowel evaluation with VCE and/or enteroscopy and radiographic testing the term occult–obscure bleeding.[4] In the setting of a positive FOBT without iron deficiency anemia, the cost effectiveness of routinely evaluating the upper GI tract in the setting of a negative colonoscopy is unclear.[2]

SUMMARY

Occult GI bleeding poses the potential for significant morbidity and mortality and can lead to significant cost for the health care system. This can affect the patient's quality-adjusted life-years and requires appropriate evaluation. It accounts for 5% to 10% of all patients presenting with GI bleeding. The evaluation is focused on finding the source of the bleeding and includes a thorough history and physical examination, upper and lower endoscopy, as well as VCE. In patients whose workup remains negative, deep enteroscopy is recommended. Of patients undergoing deep enteroscopy for occult GI bleeding a source was identified in up to 75% of patients.[4] In the 25% of patients in whom a source is not identified, further evaluation is based on the clinical picture. A trial of observation with iron supplementation may be warranted; however, there is not a clear consensus or cost analysis related to this approach. Given the high yield of deep enteroscopy, this modality has been suggested as first line in the diagnostic approach; however, owing to various limitations and concerns VCE is still recommended as the first step in the evaluation of the small intestine after traditional endoscopic approaches have not yielded a diagnosis. Furthermore, some studies have shown that, in patients with iron deficiency, up to 61% of patients with a positive test remained anemic despite receiving specific treatment. VCE was not predictive of long-term outcome, even when stratified for a change in management.[14] This area of uncertainty leaves room for further research on the long-term benefits of such an invasive approach.

ACKNOWLEDGMENTS

The author thanks Shaina M. Lynch, DO, and the Saint Francis Hospital and Medical Center Library for their contribution to this article.

REFERENCES

1. Bresci G. Occult and obscure gastrointestinal bleeding: causes and diagnostic approach in 2009. World J Gastrointest Endosc 2009;1(1):3–6.
2. Bull-Henry K, Al-Kawas FH. Evaluation of occult gastrointestinal bleeding. Am Fam Physician 2013;87(6):430–6.
3. Somsouk M, Gralnek IM, Inadomi JM. Management of obscure occult gastrointestinal bleeding: a cost-minimization analysis. Clin Gastroenterol Hepatol 2008;6(6):661–70.
4. Gerson LB, Fidler JL, Cave DR, et al. ACG clinical guideline: diagnosis and management of small bowel bleeding. Am J Gastroenterol 2015;110(9):1265–87 [quiz: 1288].
5. Rondonotti E, Marmo R, Petracchini M, et al. The American Society for Gastrointestinal Endoscopy (ASGE) diagnostic algorithm for obscure gastrointestinal bleeding: eight burning questions from everyday clinical practice. Dig Liver Dis 2013;45(3):179–85.
6. Gerson LB. Small bowel endoscopy: cost-effectiveness of the different approaches. Best Pract Res Clin Gastroenterol 2012;26(3):325–35.
7. Gerson L, Kamal A. Cost-effectiveness analysis of management strategies for obscure GI bleeding. Gastrointest Endosc 2008;68(5):920–36.
8. Weinstein MC, Stason WB. Foundations of cost-effectiveness analysis for health and medical practices. N Engl J Med 1977;296(13):716–21.
9. Gunjan D, Sharma V, Rana SS, et al. Small bowel bleeding: a comprehensive review. Gastroenterol Rep (Oxf) 2014;2(4):262–75.
10. Blecker D, Bansal M, Zimmerman RL, et al. Dieulafoy's lesion of the small bowel causing massive gastrointestinal bleeding: two case reports and literature review. Am J Gastroenterol 2001;96(3):902–5.
11. Holleran G, Hall B, Hussey M, et al. Small bowel angiodysplasia and novel disease associations: a cohort study. Scand J Gastroenterol 2013;48(4):433–8.
12. Heer M, Repond F, Hany A, et al. Acute ischaemic colitis in a female long distance runner. Gut 1987;28(7):896–9.
13. Rex DK, Johnson DA, Anderson JC, et al. American College of Gastroenterology guidelines for colorectal cancer screening 2009 [corrected]. Am J Gastroenterol 2009;104(3):739–50.
14. Holleran GE, Barry SA, Thornton OJ, et al. The use of small bowel capsule endoscopy in iron deficiency anaemia: low impact on outcome in the medium term despite high diagnostic yield. Eur J Gastroenterol Hepatol 2013;25(3):327–32.
15. Short MW, Domagalski JE. Iron deficiency anemia: evaluation and management. Am Fam Physician 2013;87(2):98–104.
16. Nissenson AR, Goodnough LT, Dubois RW. Anemia: not just an innocent bystander? Arch Intern Med 2003;163(12):1400–4.
17. Gilbert D, O'Malley S, Selby W. Are repeat upper gastrointestinal endoscopy and colonoscopy necessary within six months of capsule endoscopy in patients with obscure gastrointestinal bleeding? J Gastroenterol Hepatol 2008;23(12):1806–9.
18. Filippone A, Cianci R, Milano A, et al. Obscure and occult gastrointestinal bleeding: comparison of different imaging modalities. Abdom Imaging 2012; 37(1):41–52.

19. Marmo R, Rotondano G, Rondonotti E, et al. Capsule enteroscopy vs. other diagnostic procedures in diagnosing obscure gastrointestinal bleeding: a cost-effectiveness study. Eur J Gastroenterol Hepatol 2007;19(7):535–42.

20. Shishido T, Oka S, Tanaka S, et al. Diagnostic yield of capsule endoscopy vs. double-balloon endoscopy for patients who have undergone total enteroscopy with obscure gastrointestinal bleeding. Hepatogastroenterology 2012;59(116): 955–9.

21. Albert JG, Nachtigall F, Wiedbrauck F, et al. Minimizing procedural cost in diagnosing small bowel bleeding: comparison of a strategy based on initial capsule endoscopy versus initial double-balloon enteroscopy. Eur J Gastroenterol Hepatol 2010;22(6):679–88.

The Role of Esophagogastroduodenoscopy Surveillance for Patients with Barrett Esophagus

 CrossMark

Kerri Palamara, MD

KEYWORDS

- Barrett esophagus • Surveillance • Esophagogastroduodenoscopy • GERD
- Esophageal adenocarcinoma

KEY POINTS

- Barrett esophagus (BE) is a precursor to esophageal adenocarcinoma (EAC), but malignant transformation of dysplastic epithelium is rare.
- Patients with BE should be managed with proton pump inhibitors (PPIs) to control symptoms.
- Elderly white men with chronic gastroesophageal reflux disease (GERD) are at highest risk of BE and progression to EAC.
- Patients with BE and evidence of dysplasia on endoscopy should undergo routine surveillance according to the major gastroenterological society guidelines.

INTRODUCTION

GERD affects 40% of the general population at some point in their lives, and up to 20% of US adults report symptoms on a weekly basis.[1–3] Patients with GERD are at risk for barrett esophagus. BE is a metaplastic change in the lining of the esophageal mucosa from its normal squamous epithelium to specialized, columnar intestinal epithelium.[2–5] BE affects 5% to 6% of the average population (approximately 3 million people diagnosed annually in the United States) and up to 25% of the elderly population.[6,7] Although the overall risk for esophageal adenocarcinoma is low (26 cases per 1 million in general US population), its incidence is on the rise in Western populations, with a 300% increase since the 1970s.[4,8] Most patients with EAC present symptomatically at a stage associated with few curative interventions available and a poor prognosis. The 5-year survival rate of EAC is less than 10% and this number has not been affected by current screening and surveillance efforts.[2,8]

BE is diagnosed and monitored through endoscopy, using visual and histologic criteria, and then characterized by length and severity. First, visualization of salmon-colored

55 Fruit Street, Gray 7-730, Boston, MA 02114, USA
E-mail address: kpalamara@partners.org

Med Clin N Am 100 (2016) 1057–1064
http://dx.doi.org/10.1016/j.mcna.2016.04.014   medical.theclinics.com
0025-7125/16/$ – see front matter © 2016 Elsevier Inc. All rights reserved.

columnar epithelium in the normally white to light pink-colored tubular esophagus suggests proximal displacement of the squamocolumnar junction.[2] Second, biopsy of the tubular esophagus confirms the presence of columnar intestinal epithelium, typically containing goblet cells. If the length of the displaced squamocolumnar junction is longer than 3 cm, it is considered long-segment BE (LSBE) and shorter than 3 cm is considered short-segment BE (SSBE).[4]

EAC is thought to arise from BE through progressive dysplasia. This association raises concern for the need for screening and surveillance of patients with chronic GERD and BE to identify those at risk for progression to EAC. Although at first glance this seems logical, the utility, efficacy, and cost of such an approach must be considered. Patients with BE have a decreased quality of life compared with the general population due to inappropriately high level of fear for their risk of progression to cancer, unnecessary testing and visits, and increased life insurance premiums. In 1 study, patients diagnosed with BE experienced a 100% increase in life-insurance premiums compared with their age-matched and gender-matched controls, and some were unable to obtain insurance at all after diagnosis with BE.[9,10]

DEVELOPMENT OF BARRETT ESOPHAGUS AND ESOPHAGEAL ADENOCARCINOMA

GERD is thought to progress to BE through frequent, severe, and/or long-term exposure to acid and bile reflux. This reflux alters the normal squamous epithelium of the esophagus, which is replaced with columnar epithelium.[1,2,5] Although BE is a precursor to EAC, most patients with BE do not progress past nondysplastic or low-dysplastic disease.[2,11] The yearly esophageal cancer risk for patients with GERD who are 50 years or older is only 0.04%, and the risk of progression from BE to EAC is only 0.5% per patient year.[2,4,6]

Risk factors for the development and progression of BE and EAC include onset of symptoms before age 30, history of severe GERD symptoms, and greater than 20 cumulative years of exposure (**Fig. 1**).[1,4] The use of the term, *alarm symptoms*, describes the symptoms a patient may experience as this progression occurs. These alarm symptoms include dysphagia, anemia, weight loss, bleeding, and recurrent vomiting.

Chronic acid exposure increases the risk for BE and the subsequent segment length and severity of BE. For reasons that are not understood, men are in the highest risk group, accounting for 80% of cases of EAC. To give some perspective, rates of EAC in women are equivalent to the prevalence of breast cancer diagnoses in men.[3] In particular, elderly white men seem at the highest risk. Elderly patients are at high risk due to increased time for symptom exposure as well as a high frequency of atypical symptoms, thought to be due to less sensation to the typical heartburn symptoms of reflux.[12] Obesity is associated with increased GERD symptoms and erosive esophagitis, due to the increased risk of reflux and hiatal hernia in patients with an elevated body mass index (BMI). Patients with central obesity in particular are at an increased risk of BE due to elevated intragastric pressure.[2–4] Alcohol use and smoking have also been suggested risk factors for development of esophageal adenocarcinoma, but more recent data have been conflicting.[1,2,6,13,14]

In summary, elderly white men with chronic GERD symptoms, hiatal hernia, and elevated BMI are at greatest risk for developing severe BE and progression to EAC. Although having ever used a PPI is thought to be a risk factor for BE, one group excluded from this risk are those on a PPI due to history of *Helicobacter pylori*. Several studies have found a protective effect of prior *H pylori* infection and BE, which is not thought to be linked solely to adequate treatment of *H pylori* infection.[1,2]

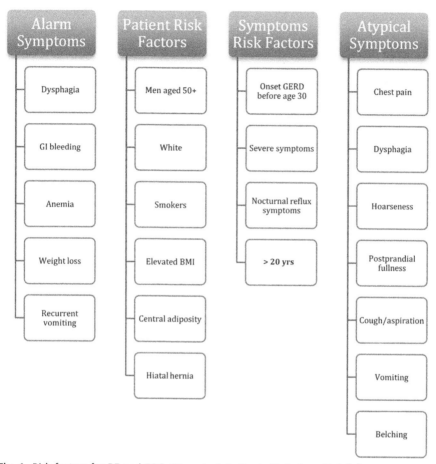

Fig. 1. Risk factors for BE and EAC. GI, gastrointestinal. (*Data from* Refs.[1–4])

Endoscopic and histologic factors associated with increased risk for progression from BE to EAC include LSBE and high-grade dysplasia. Patients with LSBE are 3 times more likely to show evidence of dysplasia on biopsy than SSBE and are at higher risk of having undetected dysplasia on endoscopy.[8,15] Even more predictive is high-grade dysplasia, the presence of which increases risk of EAC greater than 25% compared with those with no dysplasia.[4]

MANAGEMENT OF BARRETT ESOPHAGUS

The recommended treatment of BE is PPIs taken once to twice daily, 30 to 60 minutes before a meal. There is no preferred PPI based on prior studies; all have equally efficacious symptom control.[16,17] PPIs do not prevent progression to EAC in patients with BE or regress metaplastic tissue at time of treatment, but they prevent further injury and the symptoms associated with tissue injury.[2,4,18–20]

Knowing which patients with GERD will benefit from endoscopy referral is an important means to reduce overutilization. Patients with GERD who exhibit any alarm symptoms should be referred immediately for screening endoscopy. Patients with chronic reflux symptoms despite 4 to 8 weeks of maximum acid-suppression therapy should also be screened for BE. Endoscopy should not be pursued prior to 4 weeks of treatment due to the possibility of mucosal inflammation from erosive esophagitis obscuring BE.[21] In 1 study, up to 12% of SSBE was missed due to severe EE.[11,22] If symptoms persist despite initial negative endoscopy, it is reasonable to pursue a follow-up endoscopy given high possibility for sampling error. More than 20% of patients without BE on initial endoscopy have BE on subsequent endoscopy[23] (**Box 1**).

For patients diagnosed with BE with no dysplasia seen on initial endoscopy, the 3 major gastroenterological societies in the United States (American College of Gastroenterology, American Gastroenterological Association, and the American Society for Gastrointestinal Endoscopy) recommend a repeat endoscopy within a year because dysplasia can be missed.[15] Confirmation of dysplasia should prompt enrollment into a surveillance protocol based on the findings.

Patients with nondysplastic or low-dysplastic disease should be managed symptomatically with acid-reducing treatments at the lowest effective dose. Antireflux surgery could be considered in patients who are intolerant or unresponsive to acid-suppression therapy. Although treatment typically leads to return of squamous epithelium on repeat endoscopy, risk for progression to EAC persists due to concern that small islands of metaplastic tissue may remain.[4,24–26] Therefore, these patients should undergo surveillance endoscopy based on the algorithm agreed on by the gastroenterological societies and highlighted in **Fig. 2**. Those with high-grade dysplasia should be managed with high-dose PPI twice daily, frequent surveillance, and consideration of endoscopic or surgical intervention at earliest evidence of disease progression.

SURVEILLANCE CHALLENGES AND STRATEGIES

Patients with reflux who are older than 50 years have an annual esophageal cancer incidence rate of 6500 cases for every 10 million patients.[4] No study has yet shown that screening and surveillance endoscopy programs promote early detection and decrease death from EAC, and those that have suggested benefit are limited by lead-time and length-time biases.[27,28] This is not surprising given the lack of conformity with typical disease and screening characteristics professional societies adhere to when making recommendations, as illustrated in **Fig. 3**. Despite screening and surveillance guidelines, the most common indication for upper endoscopy remains GERD, and up to 40% of the endoscopies performed in the United States are not within the recommended guidelines.[3] Fear of litigation and patient disproportionate fear of malignancy may drive this overuse.[10] Outpatient endoscopies cost $800 per

---

Box 1
Who to screen for Barrett esophagus

Endoscopy referral criteria

GERD symptoms + alarm symptoms

Persistent symptoms despite 4 to 8 weeks of maximum acid reduction therapy (twice daily PPI)

Severe erosive esophagitis (after 2 months of treatment with PPI)

History of esophageal stricture + recurrent dysphagia

Consider endoscopy

Men 50+ with chronic GERD (>5 years) + additional risk factors

Data from Shaheen N, Richter J. Barretts oesophagus. Lancet 2009;373:850–61; and Allen JI. Endoscopy for gastroesophageal reflux disease: choose wisely. Ann Intern Med 2012;157(11):827–8.

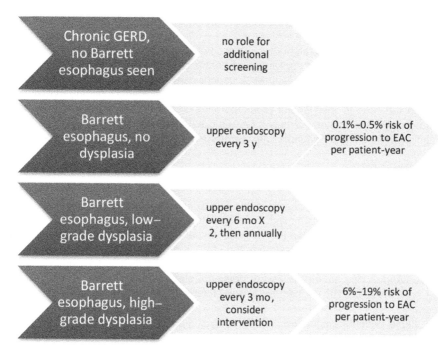

Fig. 2. Recommended BE and EAC surveillance program.

examination — $8500 if pathology and anesthesia are included — and account for more than $32 billion in health care spending annually.[29,30] The cost of loss of productivity for the patient and companion is not factored into those dollars nor is the cost of managing potential complications. Although overuse is an issue, several studies have

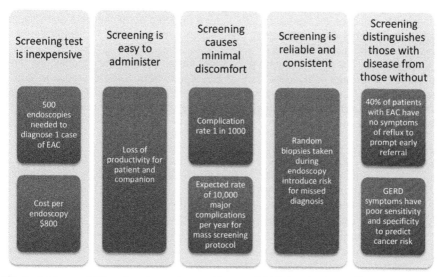

Fig. 3. Features of BE and endoscopic surveillance of EAC that limit its efficacy, cost effectiveness, and impact. (*Data from* Refs.[3,4,8])

found low rates of surveillance endoscopy in patients with BE, suggesting that under-utilization is a problem as well.[10,31]

Although the surveillance algorithm outlined in this article is a reasonable approach, caution must be taken when applying this to entire populations. One study found that only 50% of patients with frequent reflux sought care with their internist, suggesting that studies looking at rates of BE and EAC in patients referred for testing may over-estimate the risks in the general population.[32] Choosing which patients to screen based on patient and symptoms risk factors greatly reduces the risk and burden of screening while ensuring patients who warrant screening are appropriately referred.

RECOMMENDATIONS

Despite concerns that chronic reflux is a precursor of esophageal cancer, if the clinical scenario is consistent with uncomplicated GERD and there are no alarm symptoms, there is no need for a screening or diagnostic upper endoscopy. Patients with GERD should be treated with a PPI at the lowest effective dose. If symptoms persist after 8 weeks of adhering to treatment and lifestyle modifications, or if alarm symptoms develop, patients should be referred for upper endoscopy. If there is no evidence of BE on endoscopy, no further endoscopies are warranted. If erosive esophagitis is seen on a negative BE endoscopy a repeat endoscopy should be considered in 2 months.

For those patients diagnosed with BE, only a small number progress to EAC. In these patients, surveillance endoscopy should be done based on an assessment of a patient's individual risks and clinical presentation. Patients with BE and dysplasia should be monitored according to the surveillance strategies outlined by the major gastroenterological societies in the United States.

FUTURE CONSIDERATIONS

Patients with EAC are more likely to have first-degree relatives with symptoms of reflux.[5] There has been an effort to identify genetic factors associated with increased GERD symptoms and the dysplastic progression to BE and adenocarcinoma. This information could be incorporated into a more targeted screening and surveillance algorithm for better risk stratification. Identification of biomarkers for dysplastic progression is another area of focus.

Research to identify noninvasive or less invasive screening techniques has not shown improved early detection of BE, death from EAC, or reduced costs associated with screening and surveillance.[27,28,33,34] Advances in technology may serve to improve detection but may be limited by cost as well as the overall high mortality of EAC.

REFERENCES

1. Thrift AP, Kramer JR, Qureshi Z, et al. Age at onset of GERD symptoms predicts risk of Barretts esophagus. Am J Gastroenterol 2013;108(6):915–22.
2. Shaheen N, Richter J. Barretts oesophagus. Lancet 2009;373:850–61.
3. Shaheen N, Weinberg DS, Denberg T, et al, Clinical Guidelines Committee of the American College of Physicians. Upper endoscopy for gastroesophageal reflux disease: best practice advice from the clinical guidelines committee of the American College of Physicians. Ann Intern Med 2012;157(11):808–16.
4. Shaheen N, Ransohoff D. Gastroesophageal reflux, barrett esophagus, and esophageal cancer: scientific review. JAMA 2002;287:1972–81.

5. Gerson L, Lin OS. Cost-benefit analysis of capsule endoscopy compared with standard upper endoscopy for the detection of Barretts esophagus. Clin Gastroenterol Hepatol 2007;5(3):319–25.

6. Ronkainen J, Aro P, Storskrubb T, et al. Prevalence of barretts esophagus in the general population: an endoscopic study. Digestion 2000;61(1):6–13.

7. Hinojosa-Lindsey M, Arney J, Heberlig S, et al. Patients' intuitive judgments about surveillance endoscopy in Barretts esophagus: a review and application to models of decision-making. Dis Esophagus 2013;26(7):682–9.

8. Reavis KM, Morris CD, Gopal DV, et al. Laryngopharyngeal reflux symptoms better predict the presence of esophageal adenocarcinoma than typical gastroesophageal reflux symptoms. Am J Gastroenterol 2002;97(10):2524–9.

9. Shaheen NJ, Dulai GS, Ascher B, et al. Effect of a new diagnosis of Barretts esophagus on insurance status. Am J Gastroenterol 2005;100:577–80.

10. Ajumobi A, Bahiri K, Jackson C, et al. Surveillance in Barretts esophagus: an audit of practice. Dig Dis Sci 2010;55:1615–21.

11. Rodriguez S, Mattek N, Lieberman D, et al. Barretts esophagus on repeat endoscopy: should we look more than once? Am J Gastroenterol 2008;103(8):1892–7.

12. Morganstern B, Anandasabapathy S. GERD and Barretts esophagus: diagnostic and management strategies in the geriatric population. Geriatrics 2009;64(7):9–12.

13. Smith KJ, O'Brien SM, Green AC, et al. Current and past smoking significantly increase risk for Barretts esophagus. Clin Gastroenterol Hepatol 2009;7:840–8.

14. Pandeya N, Webb PM, Sadeghi S, et al. Gastrooesophageal reflux symptoms and the risks of oesophageal cancer: are the effects modified by smoking, NSAIDs or acid suppressants? Gut 2010;59:31–8.

15. Abdalla M, Dhanekula R, Greenspan M, et al. Dysplasia detection rate of confirmatory EGD in nondysplastic Barretts esophagus. Dis Esophagus 2014;27(6):505–10.

16. Dean BB, Gano AD Jr, Knight K, et al. Effectiveness of proton pump inhibitors in nonerosive reflux disease. Clin Gastroenterol Hepatol 2004;2:656–64.

17. Khan M, Santana J, Donnellan C, et al. Medical treatments in the short term management of reflux oesophagitis. Cochrane Database Syst Rev 2007;(2):CD003244.

18. Peters FT, Ganesh S, Kuipers EJ, et al. Endo-scopic regression of Barretts oesophagus during omeprazole treatment: a randomised double blind study. Gut 1999;45:489–94.

19. Cooper BT, Neumann CS, Cox MA, et al. Continuous treatment with omeprazole 20 mg daily for up to 6 years in Barretts oesophagus. Aliment Pharmacol Ther 1998;12:893–7.

20. Sharma P, Sampliner RE, Camargo E. Normalization of esophageal pH with high-dose proton pump inhibitor therapy does not result in regression of Barretts esophagus. Am J Gastroenterol 1997;92:582–5.

21. Gilani N, Gerkin RD, Ramirez FC, et al. Prevalence of Barrett's esophagus in patients with moderate to severe erosive esophagitis. World J Gastroenterol 2008;14(22):3518–22.

22. Hanna S, Rastogi A, Weston AP, et al. Detection of Barretts esophagus after endoscopic healing of erosive esophagitis. Am J Gastroenterol 2006;101:1416–20.

23. Kim SL, Waring JP, Spechler SJ, et al. Diagnostic inconsistencies in Barretts esophagus. Department of Veterans Affairs Gastroesophageal Reflux Study Group. Gastroenterology 1994;107:945–9.

24. Macey N, Le Dreau G, Volant A, et al. Adenocarcinoma of the esophagogastric junction arising after endoscopic laser photocoagulation ablation of the short segment of Barretts esophagus. Gastroenterol Clin Biol 2001;25:204–6.

25. Shand A, Dallal H, Palmer K, et al. Adenocarcinoma arising in columnar lined oesophagus following treatment with argon plasma coagulation. Gut 2001;48: 580–1.

26. Van Laethem JL, Peny MO, Salmon I, et al. Intramucosal adenocarcinoma arising un- der squamous re-epithelialisation of Barretts oesophagus. Gut 2000;46: 574–7.

27. Rubenstein JH, Sonnenberg A, Davis J, et al. Effect of a prior endoscopy on out-comes of esophageal adenocarcinoma among United States veterans. Gastroint-est Endosc 2008;68(5):849–55.

28. Rubenstein JH, Inadomi JM, Brill JV, et al. Cost utility of screening for Barretts esophagus with esophageal capsule endoscopy versus conventional upper endoscopy. Clin Gastroenterol Hepatol 2007;5(3):312–8.

29. Allen J. Endoscopy for gastroesophageal reflux disease: choose wisely. Ann Intern Med 2012;157(11):827–8.

30. Zamosky L. GERD: rising healthcare costs spark new debate, guidelines. Revised standards designed to save system money, prevent overuse of diagnos-tics. Med Econ 2013;90(1):48–54.

31. El-Serag HB, Duan Z, Hinojosa-Lindsey M, et al. Practice patterns of surveillance endoscopy in a Veterans Affairs database of 29,504 patients with Barretts esoph-agus. Gastrointest Endosc 2012;76(4):743–55.

32. Nandurkar S, Locke GR, Murray JA, et al. Rates of endoscopy and endoscopic findings among people with frequent symptoms of gastroesophageal reflux in the community. Am J Gastroenterol 2005;100(7):1459–65.

33. Atkinson M, Das A, Faulx A, et al. Ultrathin esophagoscopy in screening for Barretts esophagus at a Veterans Administration Hospital: easy access does not lead to referrals. Am J Gastroenterol 2008;103(1):92–7.

34. Lin OS, Schembre DB, Mergener K, et al. Blinded comparison of esophageal capsule endoscopy versus conventional endoscopy for a diagnosis of Barretts esophagus in patients with chronic gastroesophageal reflux. Gastrointest Endosc 2007;65(4):577–83.

The Evidence-Based Evaluation of Iron Deficiency Anemia

Eliana V. Hempel, MD, Edward R. Bollard, MD, DDS*

KEYWORDS

- Iron deficiency anemia • Microcytic anemia • Occult gastrointestinal bleed

KEY POINTS

- The identification of iron deficiency anemia and any underlying contributing comorbidities is necessary to initiate the appropriate treatment.
- In the United States, iron deficiency anemia is most prevalent in young women due to menorrhagia. In this population, a focused history, a complete blood count and a ferritin level are sufficient to confirm the diagnosis of iron deficiency anemia.
- Profoundly low mean corpuscular volume in the setting of mild anemia and a normal red cell distribution width are more suggestive of thalassemia than iron deficiency anemia and necessitate hemoglobin electrophoresis for confirmation.
- In many chronic disease states, it can be difficult to distinguish between iron deficiency anemia and anemia of chronic disease. Transferrin receptor assays and the transferrin receptor-ferritin index will help to distinguish between the two.
- Iron deficiency anemia in the elderly, even in the absence of overt gastrointestinal bleeding, necessitates endoscopic evaluation for underlying gastrointestinal malignancy.

INTRODUCTION

Anemia is of interest to the general internist, as it results in significant morbidity and mortality in a variety of patient populations. It is associated with impaired cognitive function and development in young women,[1] perinatal complications in pregnancy,[2] an increased risk of falls in the elderly[3,4] and a variety of other symptoms that affect patients' daily lives. Iron deficiency anemia (IDA) is a common cause of anemia and accounts for 50% of all cases of anemia worldwide. In the United States, IDA affects 1% to 2% of the population and is most prevalent in reproductive-aged women, affecting up to 12% of women aged 20 to 49.[5] Sufficient iron stores are required for multiple processes, including oxygen transport as part of the hemoglobin molecule, enzymatic reactions as part of the cytochrome system, and electron transport and

Disclosure Statement: The authors have nothing to disclose.
Department of Medicine, Hershey, PA, USA
* Corresponding author. 500 University Drive, PO Box 850, Hershey, PA 17033.
E-mail address: ebollard@hmc.psu.edu

Med Clin N Am 100 (2016) 1065–1075
http://dx.doi.org/10.1016/j.mcna.2016.04.015
0025-7125/16/$ – see front matter © 2016 Elsevier Inc. All rights reserved.

medical.theclinics.com

energy metabolism throughout the body.[6] Early diagnosis of IDA can prevent multiple complications and improve quality of life. However, despite the multiple complications associated with IDA, routine screening for anemia in the asymptomatic, nonpregnant population is not recommended by the US Preventive Services Task Force.[7,8]

Although iron deficiency is a common cause of anemia, there are additional potential etiologies for a reduction in the number of red blood cells or quantity of hemoglobin. Thus, on initial diagnosis of anemia, an internist must perform the appropriate evaluation to identify the cause of the anemia and subsequently select the appropriate treatment regimen. However, the process of evaluation can result in significant cost. In a nation suffering from rising health care expenditures, it is the responsibility of all physicians to do their part in decreasing this burden. Therefore, whereas identifying the underlying etiology of anemia is important, it is equally critical that we perform the evaluation in a cost-conscious manner. The purpose of this review is to suggest the most cost-effective, evidence-based assessment of IDA.

To fully understand the evaluation of IDA, we must first review the physiology of iron storage. Iron is absorbed from the diet, mainly in the small intestine, and released from stores when necessary. Free iron can be toxic to cells; therefore, it is bound to transferrin while in circulation. The transferrin-iron complex is taken up by erythroid marrow or liver parenchymal cells that express transferrin receptors. Once released from the transferrin receptor complex, iron becomes available for heme synthesis and other processes. Excess iron is bound to ferritin for storage. Hepcidin, another protein produced by the liver, is also integral in the regulation of iron stores. The physiology of hepcidin and its function in iron regulation is discussed later in this article, but it is important to note that hepcidin is increased in the setting of inflammation or iron overload and decreased in the setting of IDA.[9] It also should be noted that given the multiple mechanisms for maintenance of physiologic iron stores, true iron depletion develops over time.[10]

Case 1 Presentation

A young, otherwise healthy woman presents to the clinic with complaints of fatigue. If you were concerned for anemia as the underlying cause of her fatigue, what further information would you obtain from the patient?

As discussed previously, women of reproductive age are most commonly affected by IDA. In these and all the cases detailed later in this article, the first and most cost-conscious tool in a physician's diagnostic arsenal is the history and physical examination.

The first step in obtaining the history from this patient is to identify any other symptoms potentially attributable to IDA. A list of symptoms that occur in IDA can be seen in **Box 1**.[10,11] Next, further inquiry regarding possible etiologies of iron deficiency is warranted. These causes of IDA can be categorized into insufficient intake, malabsorption, and blood loss.

Chronic blood loss is commonly associated with menstruation and conditions involving the gastrointestinal tract. Therefore, a detailed gynecologic history as well as questions directed at symptoms of dyspepsia, melena, or hematochezia are essential. In consideration of an underlying malabsorptive state, the patient must be questioned specifically regarding symptoms related to or a personal history of inflammatory bowel disease, celiac disease, and gastrointestinal surgery.[12]

Insufficient intake of iron is rare in the United States; however, it can still occur in a variety of patients, including those with eating disorders or in individuals who follow a restricted diet, as in vegetarians and vegans. Therefore, a careful diet history can also prove useful.

Box 1
Symptoms associated with iron deficiency anemia

- Fatigue
- Dyspnea on exertion
- Dysphagia
- Pallor
- Koilonychia
- Angular stomatosis
- Cheilosis
- Glossitis
- Esophageal and pharyngeal webs
- Palpitations
- Headaches
- Tinnitus
- Taste disturbance
- Pica

Data from Clark SF. Iron deficiency anemia. Nutr Clin Pract 2008;23:128–41; and Frewin R, Henson A, Provan D. ABC of clinical haematology. Iron deficiency anemia. BMJ 1997;314:360–3.

Multiple medications, including over-the-counter preparations, can contribute both to malabsorption of iron and increased risk of bleeding. Therefore, a comprehensive medication history with particular focus on over-the-counter medications and supplements is also necessary. Specific medications that can contribute to IDA are listed in **Box 2**.

IDA itself can be a presenting symptom of other previously undiagnosed conditions. Therefore, a family history of hereditary disorders, such as inflammatory bowel disease, colorectal cancer, thalassemia, Plummer-Vinson syndrome, and bleeding disorders is necessary.

Once the history has been obtained, a thorough physical examination must be performed. Findings suggestive of IDA are listed in **Box 3**.

During your comprehensive history and physical examination, you discover that the patient described previously has been having heavy and prolonged uterine bleeding during her menstrual cycle. Due to continued suspicion for IDA, you decide to perform a laboratory evaluation. What studies would you obtain in this patient?

Box 2
Medications that may contribute to iron deficiency anemia

- Antacids
- H2 blockers
- Proton pump inhibitors
- Nonsteroidal anti-inflammatory drugs
- Aspirin
- Zinc and manganese supplements

Box 3
Physical examination findings in iron deficiency anemia

General:
- Fatigued appearing

HEENT:
- Conjunctival or lingual pallor
- Angular stomatitis
- Glossitis

Cardiovascular:
- Tachycardia
- Systolic murmur (flow murmur)

Pulmonary:
- Pulmonary edema

Abdomen:
- Hepatomegaly
- Splenomegaly

Extremities:
- Koilonychia

Skin:
- Pallor
- Poor capillary refill

Once anemia is suspected due to history and/or the physical examination, the diagnosis must be confirmed with laboratory analysis. A complete blood count (CBC) can provide not only confirmatory data but also information about the degree of the anemia and the possible etiology. Also included in a CBC are several red blood cell indices. The mean corpuscular volume (MCV) can be particularly useful with a sensitivity of 97.6% for IDA.[13,14] In IDA, the MCV is typically low with values below 80 μm^3.[15] If a microcytic, hypochromic anemia is noted on CBC, further evaluation can be limited to those conditions that result in microcytosis. However, it is important to keep in mind that although the sensitivity of MCV is high, IDA can also present with a normocytic anemia up to 40% of the time. Therefore, in the appropriate clinical context, the following evaluation may still be necessary even in the setting of normocytosis.[16] The CBC also offers the red cell distribution width (RDW). This can further help characterize microcytic anemia, as attempts at replenishing the red blood cell store in IDA would result in an increased RDW but would remain normal in thalassemia, another common cause of microcytic anemia.

Although the red blood cell indices are very useful, a peripheral smear may still be indicated in the evaluation of IDA. A peripheral smear is particularly useful in identifying features characteristic of hemolytic anemia and macrocytic anemia, such as hyper-segmented neutrophils, keratocytes, and so forth. It is less useful in the evaluation of a microcytic anemia, however, and may be avoided if microcytosis is clearly identified on the CBC.[17]

In addition to a CBC, a reticulocyte count may also prove to be useful in determining the cause of the patient's anemia. The reticulocyte count is a measure of the immature red blood cells present in circulation and reflects red cell production from the bone marrow. Due to decreased availability of substrate, the marrow cannot maintain production of reticulocytes. Therefore, the reticulocyte count is typically low in IDA.[6,18]

In this otherwise healthy young woman, the most likely etiology of microcytic anemia is IDA secondary to menstrual blood loss. The studies described later in this article may be required in the process of evaluation for IDA in this patient or others in whom you may suspect IDA. Remembering the physiology of iron transport and storage will aid in the interpretation of these values. **Table 1** includes the normal values for the studies outlined later in this article, although individual laboratory reference ranges may differ.

Serum iron levels reflect the amount of transferrin-bound iron in circulation. Total iron binding capacity (TIBC) is an indirect measure of the amount of circulating unbound transferrin. An elevated TIBC is consistent with IDA. Transferrin saturation is calculated using the following formula and is expressed as a percentage: (Iron × 100)/TIBC. With low amounts of iron available for binding to transferrin, the transferrin saturation is low in IDA, typically less than 10%.[19]

Ferritin is a reflection of the total amount of stored iron in the body. In IDA, the ferritin is typically low, with values less than 15 μg/L being highly suggestive of a diagnosis of IDA. A ferritin level of less than 45 μg/L is 85% sensitive and 92% specific for IDA. The sensitivity and specificity of ferritin once the level rises above 45 (45–100 ng/mL) decreases significantly to 9.4% and 80.0% respectively.[13,14]

Other less commonly ordered but also useful studies include protoporphyrin levels and transferrin receptor assays. Protoporphyrin functions in the pathway of heme synthesis and is a reflection of the rate of synthesis. If heme synthesis is impaired by a lack of iron, protoporphyrin builds up in the cell, resulting in elevated levels in IDA.[10]

A transferrin receptor assay reflects the amount of available transferrin receptors and is performed using enzyme-linked immunosorbent assay testing. In IDA, transferrin receptors are upregulated, resulting in elevated transferrin receptor levels. Transferrin receptor levels have been studied and shown to be an accurate marker of IDA, even in the setting of inflammation.[20] It is, therefore, especially useful in distinguishing between IDA and anemia of chronic disease (ACD), where the transferrin receptor level would be normal.[20]

Table 1
Normal values for laboratory studies

Laboratory Study	Normal Values
Hemoglobin	♂ >13 g/dL, ♀ >12 g/dL
Reticulocyte count	1%–2%
Iron	50–150 μg/dL
Ferritin	♂ 100 μg/dL, ♀ 30 μg/dL
TIBC	300–360 μg/dL
Transferrin saturation	25%–50%
Protoporphyrin	<30 μg/dL
Transferrin receptor assay	4–9 μg/L

Data from Adamson J. Iron deficiency anemia and other hypoproliferative anemias. In: Kasper D, Fauci A, Hauser S, et al, editors. Harrisons. 19th edition. New York: McGraw-Hill; 2015. p. 626–8.

Although ferritin can be a very worthwhile study in the evaluation of IDA, it also can be misleading. As an acute phase reactant, it can be elevated in the setting of infection and other chronic diseases. This may lead the interpreter away from a true diagnosis of IDA, especially in elderly patients with multiple comorbidities. In instances in which the clinical picture and the ferritin do not correlate with each other, another alternative diagnostic tool is the transferrin receptor-ferritin index. It has been studied in comparison with transferrin receptor levels alone and was found to be highly sensitive and 93% specific for the diagnosis of IDA.[21] It is calculated using the ratio of the serum transferrin receptor to the log ferritin level.[14] Ratios less than 1 are more consistent with ACD, whereas ratios greater than 2 are more suggestive of IDA.[22]

The gold standard for diagnosis of IDA is iron staining of a bone marrow aspirate. In IDA, staining would be absent or decreased. Bone marrow staining is more expensive and more invasive than the other studies previously described and is typically unnecessary.

Although the testing outlined previously is available, all of these tests may not be necessary. In an otherwise healthy woman of reproductive age, a detailed history and physical examination, CBC, and ferritin are likely sufficient to diagnose IDA.[19] If ferritin levels are nondiagnostic, serum iron, TIBC, and transferrin saturation are appropriate next steps.

Conclusion: You refer the patient for laboratory studies and confirm a diagnosis of anemia with a CBC that reveals a moderate normocytic anemia with an expanded RDW. In conjunction with the CBC, you also ordered a ferritin which returned significantly depressed. The patient is counseled on initiation of iron supplementation. Consideration is also given to the addition of oral contraceptive agents to control the source of her IDA, her menorrhagia.

Case 2 Presentation

A 25-year-old, healthy woman of Indian descent presents to the clinic after evaluation in the emergency department for right lower quadrant pain. In the process of her evaluation, she had a CBC performed that revealed a mild microcytic anemia. She was instructed to follow up with her primary care physician. She reports minimal fatigue but otherwise has no associated symptoms. You suspect thalassemia. What evaluation would you perform to distinguish between thalassemia and IDA?

Thalassemia is an autosomal recessive hemoglobinopathy that results in microcytic anemia. Beta chains are affected in beta thalassemia and those who are heterozygous for this condition are said to have beta thalassemia minor (thalassemia trait). Beta thalassemia minor can be difficult to distinguish from IDA, as they both present with mild to moderate microcytic anemias. Patients with beta thalassemia minor are typically asymptomatic and diagnosed incidentally. However, misdiagnosis of IDA in a patient with beta thalassemia minor will result in futile treatment with supplemental iron. Additionally, patients with beta thalassemia need preconception counseling to be educated on the hereditary nature of their disease. Thus, it is important to identify the correct cause of the microcytic anemia in these patients.

Findings that can aid in this distinction are the degree of microcytosis and the red cell indices. Thalassemia typically presents with profound microcytosis despite having relatively mild anemia. The MCV in a patient with thalassemia is typically less than 75 μm^3, whereas MCVs are typically depressed, but often above 80 μm^3 in IDA. Additionally, as the red blood cells are fairly uniform in thalassemia, the RDW is normal. An elevated RDW would be expected in IDA.[23,24] The red blood cell (RBC) count has been found to be most helpful in differentiating between IDA and beta thalassemia, with a sensitivity and specificity above 80%. An RBC count less than 5×10^{12}/L is consistent with IDA.[25,26] If the red cell indices support a diagnosis of thalassemia trait, the next best diagnostic test is hemoglobin electrophoresis.

Conclusion: A hemoglobin electrophoresis reveals beta thalassemia minor. She is counseled on the possibility of worsening of her anemia during pregnancy and the chances of her condition being passed on to her children.

Case 3 Presentation

A 30-year-old gentleman with a history of known Crohn disease that is well controlled presents with a longstanding history of progressive fatigue and depression. Recent blood work revealed anemia. What possible etiologies would you consider for his anemia and how might you begin his evaluation?

In the absence of obvious blood loss as a source of IDA, other diagnoses must be considered. Although this patient presents with known Crohn disease, his symptoms have been well controlled. Due to the high degree of variability in severity and presenting symptoms, other similar patients may not yet carry the diagnosis of inflammatory bowel disease (IBD) and can go untreated for prolonged periods of time. Anemia has been identified as an exceedingly common extraintestinal manifestation of IBD. IDA is the most common subtype of anemia in this population with a prevalence of 30% to 90%.[27] The high prevalence of anemia in IBD is likely secondary to 2 contributing mechanisms of iron deficiency. The intestinal inflammation likely leads to decreased absorption of iron, and the chronic bleeding associated with IBD leads to persistent losses. However, malabsorption can also lead to B12 and folate deficiency and chronic inflammatory processes can lead to ACD.

Distinguishing IDA from other causes of anemia in IBD can be challenging. Identification of the underlying etiology is nonetheless an important task, as treatment decisions depend on the type(s) of anemia involved.

ACD is another common cause of anemia. It is important to understand the suspected underlying physiology to be able to distinguish between ACD and IDA. In addition to inflammatory diseases, such as IBD, ACD also can be caused by chronic infections and malignancy. The pathophysiology of ACD is still not well understood and is likely multifactorial. One of the main culprit proteins identified in ACD is hepcidin. Hepatocytes produce hepcidin and it functions in iron metabolism. Hepcidin binds to and blocks ferroportin. Ferroportin is required to access stored iron. Interleukin (IL)-6, an inflammatory cytokine, is increased in the setting of inflammation. IL-6 leads to the increased production of hepcidin, thus resulting in inhibited access to iron stores. In contrast, it is suspected that hepcidin is downregulated in IDA, allowing for release of stored iron and increased iron absorption.[9]

Additionally, there is some evidence to suggest that iron absorption is also affected by chronic inflammation. The increase in inflammatory cytokines has been implicated in suppression of RBC production in the bone marrow. RBC longevity is also affected by ACD, again likely due to inflammatory cytokine-mediated activation of macrophages.[9,22,28]

Unfortunately, the laboratory evaluation detailed previously may not be useful in distinguishing IDA from ACD. Nutritional deficiencies associated with chronic malabsorption can decrease albumin levels. Hypoalbuminemia is associated with low transferrin levels. Therefore, transferrin levels may not be accurate in IDA associated with IBD. Additionally, ferritin, as an acute phase reactant, is often elevated in chronic inflammation and is also unreliable. In this setting, soluble transferrin receptor assays and transferrin receptor-ferritin indices will be most useful.[27]

Impaired absorption and inflammatory states are not limited to IBD alone. Other gastrointestinal conditions that can result in malabsorption include celiac disease and post resection or post gastric bypass states.[16] As noted previously, proper identification of the underlying etiology is important, as it dictates treatment. In celiac disease, for example, untreated disease can lead to persistent alterations of the duodenal mucosa that persistently impair iron absorption. Therefore, even if IDA is correctly diagnosed, lack of treatment of the underlying condition can lead to refractory anemia.

Conclusion: In the process of evaluation of this gentleman's anemia, a ferritin was obtained and was nondiagnostic. Subsequently, a transferrin receptor assay was performed and was found to be elevated. The transferrin receptor-ferritin index was greater than 2, confirming a diagnosis of IBD-associated IDA. Due to concern for intolerance and poor absorption of oral iron in the setting of IBD, iron supplementation intravenously was initiated and the patient's symptoms gradually improved.

Case 4 Presentation

A 62-year-old otherwise healthy gentleman presents to the clinic with complaints of dyspnea on exertion and palpitations. He does not disclose any additional symptoms. With the exception of mild pallor, his physical examination is normal. A CBC is obtained due to concern for anemia and reveals mild anemia. What additional workup would you consider in this case?

In men and postmenopausal women, IDA is associated with gastrointestinal lesions 50% to 70% of the time.[14,29] In a prospective study performed with the goal of assessing a guideline-based approach to the evaluation of anemia, the findings revealed a significant rise in the number of serious gastrointestinal lesions identified once a diagnosis of IDA was established. In this study, of the 100 patients evaluated with upper and lower endoscopy, 62 patients were found to have a likely culprit lesion. Because IDA can be the presenting symptom of underlying gastrointestinal malignancy in patients older than 50, further evaluation with endoscopy is indicated. If there are no signs of overt bleeding, such as melena or hematochezia, it is reasonable to initiate evaluation with a fecal occult blood test, although a negative fecal occult blood test does not preclude the need for further endoscopic evaluation. Positive fecal occult blood tests in combination with localized gastrointestinal symptoms have been found to correlate strongly with bleeding lesions at the predicted site.

Signs and symptoms associated with identification of a suspect lesion include age older than 50 years, male gender, recent nonsteroidal anti-inflammatory drug use and more significant anemia (hemoglobin <9 g/dL).[30,31] This suggests that we may be able to direct our initial endoscopic evaluation to the location of symptoms.[32] If an upper endoscopy is indicated by the clinical presentation and a suspect lesion is identified, the patient likely does not require further evaluation with a colonoscopy, assuming the patient is up to date on current recommendations for colorectal cancer screening. This would result in not only decrease in unnecessary resource utilization but also limit the risks associated with avoidable procedures.

In an otherwise asymptomatic patient with IDA, especially elderly patients in whom the risk of malignancy is high, it is reasonable to initiate workup with a colonoscopy. In the setting of a negative colonoscopy, subsequent upper endoscopy is necessary.[32]

If endoscopic evaluation is unrevealing and anemia is not severe, oral iron supplementation and monitoring are acceptable. However, 5% of tumors resulting in IDA are missed due to improper bowel preparation, operator variability, and other factors affecting reliability of colonoscopy. Therefore, if anemia and symptoms are persistent despite a negative endoscopic evaluation, repeat upper endoscopy and colonoscopy are indicated.

If, despite multiple endoscopic evaluations, a lesion is still not identified and the patient has persistent anemia, the lesion is likely located in the small bowel. Evaluation of the small bowel can be challenging. The options for investigation include video capsule endoscopy (VCE) and single or double balloon enteroscopy (SBE). VCE is less invasive but is limited in that it can still fail to identify the lesion, and if a lesion is identified and treatment is necessary, enteroscopy is still required. In a meta-analysis that reviewed VCE versus other forms of small bowel evaluation, the yield of VCE for a culprit lesion was higher than that of SBE and small bowel barium radiography. This particular meta-analysis did not find a statistically significant difference in the identification of malignant lesions compared with SBE. Nevertheless, VCE information is valuable, as vascular or inflammatory lesions can still be major contributors in the development of IDA and may require treatment.[33]

Another randomized study investigated VCE versus push enteroscopy as first-line evaluation of obscure gastrointestinal bleeding identified by either overt bleeding or chronic IDA with a negative workup. This study reported that VCE did not fail to identify the bleeding lesion in any cases, whereas SBE failed to identify a lesion that was subsequently identified with VCE in 26% of patients.[34]

SBE affords the ability to both identify and treat the lesion simultaneously and has previously been shown to successfully locate the likely bleeding lesions in 53% of cases of obscure gastrointestinal bleeding.[32] However, in addition to the higher rate of missed lesions, it is significantly more invasive, can be technically difficult, and can result in postprocedural complications. Although the yield of VCE has been variable in the multiple studies performed to compare it with other modalities, the risk/benefit ratio is in favor of initiating evaluation with VCE.[35–42]

Conclusion: Despite his lack of overt gastrointestinal bleeding, due to his age and subsequent laboratory findings suggestive of IDA, this patient was referred for colonoscopy. He was found to have two, 2-cm adenomatous polyps that were successfully removed. He was scheduled for follow-up colonoscopy.

In summary, IDA is a common disease that the internist will encounter regularly. It can take many forms and has multiple possible etiologies. A detailed history and thorough physical examination are both cost-effective and valuable. Based on diagnostic information obtained in the history and physical, further laboratory evaluation can be limited to the studies with the highest yield, depending on the clinical scenario. Appropriate identification of IDA and any underlying contributing pathologies is critical in the management of this condition.

REFERENCES

1. Murray-Kolb L, Beard J. Iron treatment normalizes cognitive function in young women. Am J Clin Nutr 2007;85:778–87.
2. Rasmussen K. Is there a causal relationship between iron deficiency or iron-deficiency anemia and weight at birth, length of gestation and perinatal mortality? J Nutr 2001;131:590S–603S.
3. Pennix BW, Pluijm SM, Lips P, et al. Late-life anemia is associated with increased risk of recurrent falls. J Am Geriatr Soc 2005;53:2106–11.
4. Dhamarajan TS, Avula S, Norkus EP. Anemia increases risk for falls in hospitalized older adults: an evaluation of falls in 362 hospitalized, ambulatory, long-term care, and community patients. J Am Med Dir Assoc 2007;8:e9–15.
5. Centers for Disease Control and Prevention (CDC). Iron deficiency–United States, 1999-2000. MMWR Morb Mortal Wkly Rep 2002;51:897–9.

6. Adamson J. Iron deficiency anemia and other hypoproliferative anemias. In: Kasper D, Fauci A, Hauser S, et al, editors. Harrisons. 19th edition. McGraw-Hill; 2015. Available at: http://accessmedicine.mhmedical.com.medjournal.hmc.psu.edu:2048/content.aspx?sectionid=79731112&bookid=1130&Resultclick=2&q=iron%20anemia. Accessed November, 2015.

7. McCarthy M. Evidence for iron deficiency screening "inadequate" US panel concludes. BMJ 2015;350:1841.

8. Cantor A, Bougatsos C, Dana T, et al. Routine iron supplementation and screening for iron deficiency anemia in pregnancy: a systematic review for the U.S. Preventative Services Task Force. Ann Intern Med 2015;162:566–76.

9. Camaschella C. Iron-deficiency anemia. N Engl J Med 2015;372:1832–43.

10. Clark SF. Iron deficiency anemia. Nutr Clin Pract 2008;23:128–41.

11. Frewin R, Henson A, Provan D. ABC of clinical haematology. Iron deficiency anemia. BMJ 1997;314:360–3.

12. Bermeja J, Garcia-Lopez S. A guide to diagnosis of iron deficiency and iron deficiency anemia in digestive diseases. World J Gastroenterol 2009;15:4638–43.

13. Ioannou GN, Spector J, Scott K, et al. Prospective evaluation of a clinical guideline for the diagnosis and management of IDA. Am J Med 2002;113:281–7.

14. Guyatt GH, Patterson C, Ali M, et al. Diagnosis of iron deficiency anemia in the elderly. Am J Med 1990;88:205–9.

15. Killip S, Bennett J, Chambers M. Iron deficiency anemia. Am Fam Physician 2007; 75:671–8.

16. Johnson-Wimbley T. Diagnosis and management of iron deficiency anemia in the 21st century. Therap Adv Gastroenterol 2011;4:177–84.

17. Bain B. Diagnosis from the blood smear. N Engl J Med 2005;353:498–507.

18. Means. Iron deficiency anemia. Hematology 2013;18:305–6.

19. Punnonen K, Irjala K, Rajamaki A. Serum transferrin receptor and its ratio to serum ferritin in the diagnosis of iron deficiency. Blood 1997;89:1052–7.

20. Cullis J. Diagnosis and management of anemia of chronic disease: current status. BMJ 2011;154:289–300.

21. Provan D, O'Shaughnessy D. Recent advances in hematology. BMJ 1999;318: 991–4.

22. Gomollon F, Gisbert J. Current management of IDA in IBD: a practical guide. Drugs 2013;73:1761–70.

23. Nemeth E, Ganz T. Anemia of inflammation. Hematol Oncol Clin North Am 2014; 28:671–81.

24. Guyatt GH, Oxman AD, Ali M, et al. Laboratory diagnosis of iron deficiency anemia: an overview. J Gen Intern Med 1992;7:423.

25. Majid S, Salih M, Wasaya R, et al. Predictors of gastrointestinal lesions on endoscopy in iron deficiency anemia without gastrointestinal symptoms. BMC Gastroenterol 2008;8:52.

26. James M, Chen C, Goddard W, et al. Risk factors for GI malignancy in patients with iron-deficiency anaemia. Eur J Gastroenterol Hepatol 2005;17:1197–203.

27. Descamps C, Schmit A, Van Gossum A. "Missed" upper GI tract lesions may explain "occult" bleeding. Endoscopy 1999;31:452–5.

28. Triester S, Leighton JA, Leontiadis GI, et al. A meta-analysis of the yield of capsule endoscopy compared to other diagnostic modalities in patients with obscure gastrointestinal bleeding. Am J Gastroenterol 2005;100:2407–18.

29. De Leusse A, Vahedi K, Edery J, et al. Capsule endoscopy or push enteroscopy for first line exploration of obscure gastrointestinal bleeding? Gastroenterology 2007;132:855–62.

30. Gupta R, Reddy D. Capsule endoscopy: current status in obscure gastrointestinal bleeding. World J Gastroenterol 2007;13:4551–3.
31. Van Vraken M. Evaluation of microcytosis. Am Fam Physician 2010;82:1117–22.
32. Rimon E. Diagnosis of iron deficiency anemia in the elderly by transferrin receptor-ferritin index. Arch Intern Med 2002;162:445–9.
33. Powers J, Buchanan G. Diagnosis and management of iron deficiency anemia. Hematol Oncol Clin North Am 2014;28:729–45.
34. Ott C, Scholmerich J. Extraintestinal manifestations and complications in IBD. Nat Rev Gastroenterol Hepatol 2013;10:585–95.
35. Cook JD. Diagnosis and management of iron deficiency anemia. Best Pract Res Clin Haematol 2005;18:319–32.
36. Thomas D, Hinchliffe R, Briggs C, et al. Guideline for the laboratory diagnosis of functional iron deficiency. Br J Haematol 2013;161:639–48.
37. Rockey D, Cello J. Evaluation of the gastrointestinal tract in patients with iron-deficiency anemia. N Engl J Med 1992;329:1691–5.
38. Mast A, Blinder M, Lu Q, et al. Clinical utility of the reticulocyte hemoglobin content in the diagnosis of iron deficiency. Blood 2002;99:1489–91.
39. Cao A, Galanello R. Beta-thalassemia. Genet Med 2010;12:61–76.
40. Olivieri N. The beta-thalassemias. N Engl J Med 1999;341:99–109.
41. Beyan C, Kaptan K, Ifran A. Predictive value of discrimination indices in differential diagnosis of iron deficiency anemia and beta-thalassemia trait. Eur J Haematol 2007;78:524–6.
42. Okan V, Cigiloglu A, Cifci S, et al. Red cell indices and functions differentiation patients with beta-thalassemia trait from those with iron deficiency anemia. J Int Med Res 2009;37:25–30.

Indications and Usefulness of Common Injections for Nontraumatic Orthopedic Complaints

 CrossMark

Robert K. Cato, MD

KEYWORDS

- Joint injections • Steroid injections • Corticosteroids • Tendinopathy • Arthritis

KEY POINTS

- Corticosteroid injections (CSIs) are commonly used in the treatment of painful musculo-skeletal conditions, despite a lack of consensus in the literature of the true usefulness.
- Any benefits of CSIs are of modest magnitude and short lived, on the order of a few weeks. There are no long-term benefits, and no change in future need for surgical intervention.
- Hyaluronic acid injections to treat knee osteoarthritis are widely used, although the benefits are modest and short term, and the cost is high.
- Injections for treatment of painful musculoskeletal conditions are generally safe and well tolerated, although in some circumstances there are suggestions of long-term deleterious outcomes.

INTRODUCTION

Pain related to various musculoskeletal (MS) conditions is a common patient complaint, and one that is often difficult to remedy. In addition to oral analgesics and physical therapy, local injections (most commonly of corticosteroid [CS]) are a common intervention and have been for decades. However, in most cases, the literature is full of poor-quality studies, making the true utility of these injections questionable. This article reviews some of the literature studying these injections with the goal of providing clinicians the information to make evidence-based, high-value choices.

OSTEOARTHRITIS OF THE KNEE

Osteoarthritis of the knee is a common problem in Western societies, especially in the elderly, and is one of the biggest causes of disability.[1] There is no cure, and joint

Disclosure: The author has nothing to disclose.
Penn Presbyterian Medical Center, 51 North 29th Street, Medical Arts Building, Suite 102, Philadelphia, PA 19104, USA
E-mail address: Robert.Cato@uphs.upenn.edu

Med Clin N Am 100 (2016) 1077–1088
http://dx.doi.org/10.1016/j.mcna.2016.04.007
0025-7125/16/$ – see front matter © 2016 Elsevier Inc. All rights reserved.

replacement surgery is expensive and carries significant risks. Therefore, treatment is focused on pain relief interventions and maintaining function. Injection therapy (notably CSs and hyaluronic acid derivatives) are widely used. Various other modalities have been studied in this regard, including exercise therapy, braces, and oral medications, and these must be kept in context for comparison purposes.

Corticosteroid Injections for Osteoarthritis of the Knee: Efficacy

Corticosteroid injections (CSIs) have been used in osteoarthritis of the knee since the 1950s, and there have been numerous studies, many of them small and with significant methodological flaws that limit the interpretation of the results. For example, many studies did not use validated pain scales, and frequently the severity of osteoarthritis was not reported. The studies that are the most useful are double blinded and placebo controlled, and use validated measures of improvement, such as validated pain scales and objective functional measures.

A meta-analysis by Arroll and Goodyear-Smith[2] in 2004 found 10 studies of reasonably good quality and determined that intra-articular steroid injections led to statistically significant improvements in pain, stiffness, and function at 1 week and 2 weeks but not at various later end points, up to 6 months. When they combined the 2 studies that followed patients for 24 weeks, they found a statistically significant improvement compared with baseline, but no difference compared with placebo. The meta-analysis also suggested that higher doses of steroids, such as 40 mg of methylprednisolone or 40 mg of triamcinolone, are superior to the lower doses used in some studies.

A later systematic review was done by Hepper and colleagues[3] in 2009, in which 6 randomized placebo-controlled studies were examined. They used a 100-point analog pain scale, and all 6 of these studies showed a significant benefit from steroid injection at both 1 and 2 weeks, with a reduction in pain of about 50% (20–33 points on the scale). Note that 3 of 5 studies also showed a benefit to placebo at these time points, but to a smaller scale (7%–20%, up to 20 points on the analog scale). All studies showed that the steroid injection was superior in efficacy to the placebo, which was usually saline and/or lidocaine. Similar to the Arroll and Goodyear-Smith[2] meta-analysis, the incremental benefit of the steroid injections seemed to fade after 2-weeks.

Bannuru and colleagues[4] in 2015 did a network meta-analysis and systematic review to compare the efficacy of various interventions in treating osteoarthritis of the knee. They concluded that intra-articular CSIs were superior to oral placebo, injected placebo, and oral nonsteroidal antiinflammatory medications in the short term. They also found that injected placebo was superior to oral placebo. However, they commented on the wide variety of studies and the inconsistency in the literature, and stated that further studies were warranted.

The aforementioned studies were all limited to the effects of 1 injection, but it is possible that repeated injections may have cumulative benefits over time. Raynauld and colleagues[5] studied 68 patients with moderate osteoarthritis of the knee and randomized them in double-blind fashion to receive either triamcinolone 40 mg or saline every 3 months for 2 years (total of 8 injections). They found borderline significant benefit to the steroid injections at 1 year in night pain, as well as a general trend toward improvement in many other measures, but these differences over time were small and did not reach statistical significance in this small study. At 2 years, there were no differences and all trends had disappeared.

A recent Cochrane systematic review[6] concluded that the data for intra-articular steroid injection utility in the treatment of osteoarthritis remains overall very poor, but that there is probably a moderate benefit of corticosteroid injection for 2 weeks, a small benefit at 8 weeks, and little or no benefit at 12 to 26 weeks.

Corticosteroid Injections for Osteoarthritis of the Knee: Safety

In general, intra-articular steroid injections of the knee are very low risk. Typical side effects of CSs, such as transient worsening of diabetes control, are mild and self-limited. Local reactions such as pain, redness, and swelling may occur. Very rarely injection can lead to infections. One concern that is often discussed is possible hastening of cartilage wasting and worsening of osteoarthritis as a result of repeated steroid injections. In the Raynauld and colleagues[5] study mentioned earlier, patients received a total of 8 injections over the course of 2 years, and no deleterious effects were noted between the placebo saline and CSI groups. This study included an analysis of fluoroscopically determined joint space.

Corticosteroid Injections for Osteoarthritis of the Knee: Cost

$50 to $200 per injection, including injection charge and medication.

Corticosteroid Injections for Osteoarthritis of the Knee: Conclusions

Despite the variable results and overall poor data quality, it seems that CSIs are modestly helpful in some patients with knee osteoarthritis in the short term, but do not seem to be helpful in the long term. They are generally safe and well tolerated, and, as long as the patient is clear on the expectations, may help in the management of pain and dysfunction in patients with osteoarthritis of the knee. This advice is in keeping with the American College of Rheumatology 2012 guidelines,[7] although the American Academy of Orthopedic Surgeons 2013 guideline could not recommend for or against the use of CSIs for treatment of osteoarthritis of the knee because of inconclusive evidence.[8,9]

Intra-articular Injection of Hyaluronic Acids in Knee Osteoarthritis: Efficacy

Hyaluronic acid is a naturally occurring substance found in synovial fluid, and is thought to act as a lubricant and shock absorber. Several preparations of varying molecular weights have been developed for intra-articular injection in patients with osteoarthritis of the knee, and are usually termed viscosupplementation.[1] When assessing efficacy, there are many conflicting results and many studies that lacked proper placebo groups or had other methodological flaws. Some studies found no effect on pain and function, whereas others found a positive effect, including one that had a surprisingly large reduction in pain on visual analog scales, with a reduction of 30 points on a 100-point scale. To address these discrepancies, several systematic reviews and meta-analyses have been performed.

Arrich and colleagues[10] found 22 articles that included quantification of pain scales, and on systematic review and meta-analysis there was a mean reduction in visual analog score pain scales of 3 to 7 points (out of 100) at various time points out to 6 months. There was high heterogeneity among trials, and many did not include intention-to-treat analysis, or failed to have blinding. They concluded that the aggregate data are flawed overall, preventing firm conclusions, but there may be a small benefit, of questionable clinical significance, to hyaluronic acid injections. Rutjes and colleagues[11] did a more recent systematic review and meta-analysis, and found 71 trials that showed a benefit to hyaluronate injections. However, they also uncovered unpublished studies that did not show benefit, and concluded that, overall, based on the available data, there is a small clinically insignificant benefit.

In contrast, a Cochrane Review in 2006 concluded that "viscosupplementation is an effective treatment for OA [osteoarthritis] of the knee with beneficial effects: on pain, function and patient global assessment; and at different post injection periods but especially at the 5 to 13 week post injection period."[12] The review pointed out the wide variability in responses seen in the different studies and the use of different products. The investigators were not able to comment on the benefits of one product compared with another except that a trend existed favoring the higher-molecular-weight substances compared with lower-weight substances.

The American Academy of Orthopedic Surgery revised its guidelines in 2013, stating that intra-articular hyaluronic acid is no longer recommended as a method of treatment of patients with symptomatic osteoarthritis of the knee. They cited a lack of clinically meaningful benefits in meta-analysis.

Intra-articular Injection of Hyaluronic Acids in Knee Osteoarthritis: Safety

There are no studies showing any long-term risks with intra-articular injections of hyaluronic acids, although this has been poorly studied. The injections have a statistically significant increased risk of local adverse effects compared with placebo (Relative Risk = 2), primarily in the form of flares of osteoarthritis that are thought to be caused by inflammatory reaction to the local injection. In some patients this is severe and function limiting, but reversible.

Intra-articular Injection of Hyaluronic Acids in Knee Osteoarthritis: Cost

The cost of these injections can vary widely depending on the product selected and the physician charge. In addition, depending on the product, the number needed can range from 1 to 5 injections. However, costs seem to be between $1200 and $1500.

Intra-articular Injection of Hyaluronic Acids in Knee Osteoarthritis: Conclusion

The efficacy of hyaluronates in the treatment of osteoarthritis remains in question, although most studies suggest either no clinically significant benefit or a modest benefit, without major harms, but at significant cost. These injections may be used, but only in specific circumstances after other, more proven treatments have been used.

SHOULDER PAIN (IMPINGEMENT SYNDROME)

CSIs in patients with shoulder pain have been used for more than 50 years. However, the data on their efficacy are conflicting and variable. Many studies are poorly designed, lacking validated pain scales and placebo controls. Another major problem with the literature on this subject is the wide variety of causes of shoulder pain, including rotator cuff tears, rotator cuff tendinopathy, acromioclavicular joint arthritis, glenohumeral joint arthritis, subacromial bursitis, and adhesive capsulitis. Many studies do not specify the cause, or do not show how the underlying cause was determined. To complicate matters further, the presence of a finding on imaging does not necessarily prove the cause of the problem, because many patients have asymptomatic rotator cuff disease or shoulder arthritis. This article focuses on the use of CSI for treatment of the common impingement syndrome conditions, including bursitis and rotator cuff tendinopathy.

Corticosteroid Injection for Shoulder Impingement Syndrome: Efficacy

Koester and colleagues[13] did a systematic review of the literature as of 2007, assessing the efficacy of subacromial injections in the treatment of rotator cuff disease. They found 9 randomized placebo-controlled studies that specifically studied patients with rotator cuff disease, either tendinopathy alone or with partial cuff tears. All of the studies had small numbers of subjects, all less than 100. Some of the studies included only patients with short periods of symptoms (several weeks), and others studied patients with chronic (>6 months) pain. All of the studies measured pain, either on visual analog scales or by other means, as well as range of motion. Of the 9 studies, only 4 found a statistically significant reduction in pain scales (up to 24 weeks), and 3 showed an improvement in range of motion. However, the clinical significance of these changes was questionable overall, especially with range-of-motion improvements, which tended to be small (range, 5°–10°). The investigators concluded that, overall, the benefit of CSIs in rotator cuff disease is not supported by the literature.

In contrast, Arroll and Goodyear-Smith[14] did a meta-analysis of CSIs for painful shoulders and found a benefit to subacromial injection overall, potentially out to 9 months. This analysis used a dichotomous variable of improvement versus no improvement, and calculated a number needed to treat (NNT) of 2 to 3 overall. However, this review did not limit the type of shoulder disorder, and there was a high degree of heterogeneity among the studies (which places these conclusions in significant doubt overall).

In one of the better designed trials, Alvarez and colleagues[15] compared subacromial injections of betamethasone plus xylocaine with xylocaine alone (control group) in 58 patients with up to 6 months of symptoms related to rotator cuff tendinopathy or partial cuff tear. Of note, these patients were randomized and blinded, and had already failed a more conservative approach of nonsteroidal antiinflammatory medications plus physical therapy. At various time points out to 6 months, a modest improvement in symptoms occurred in both groups, but there was no significant difference between the two groups overall in shoulder function, pain, or quality-of-life measures.

In addition, in a recent study Rhon and colleagues[16] compared subacromial CSIs (up to 3 in total, spaced 1 month apart) with 3 weeks of manual physical therapy in 100 randomized patients with shoulder impingement syndrome. Both groups had a significant 50% improvement in SPADI (shoulder pain and disability index) scores compared with baseline at all points in the study (1–12 months). However, the two groups did not differ in efficacy, and the injection group had more health care interactions, and twice as many subjects returned throughout the year for injection compared with the physical therapy group. However, both groups had improvement compared with baseline, and the investigators concluded that both of these interventions offer benefit to patients with impingement syndrome.

Corticosteroid Injection for Shoulder Impingement Syndrome: Safety

In the various randomized studies, no significant complications were reported apart from local pain and redness. Specifically, there were no reports of tendon rupture. There are case reports of septic bursitis, usually with *Staphylococcus aureus*, following subacromial injection,[17] but this is a rare complication. Worsening of glycemic control may occur in patients given CSIs, although generally this is a self-limited issue. More importantly, concerns have been raised about the effects of CSIs on the rotator cuff tendons, and various animal studies have shown significant softening and other changes to the tendons with repeat injections. One study found a higher rate of cuff repair failure in patients who had more than 3 subacromial CSIs preoperatively, although this has not been replicated elsewhere and is not definitive.[18]

Corticosteroid Injection for Shoulder Impingement Syndrome: Cost

Total cost for CSI of the shoulder (medication and physician fee) can vary, but generally ranges from $50 to $200.

Corticosteroid Injection for Shoulder Impingement Syndrome: Conclusions

In patients with impingement syndrome, including subacromial bursitis and rotator cuff tendinopathy or partial tears, CSI seems to have limited benefit that is not necessarily clinically significant for most patients. On the whole, CSI does not seem to be superior to physical therapy in the long term, although individual responses vary. There are no common significant risks. CSI is likely to remain an option for treatment of impingement syndrome, especially in patients with severe pain or who have not responded to other measures.

LATERAL EPICONDYLITIS (EPICONDYLALGIA)

Lateral epicondylitis is a common condition characterized by pain at the lateral epicondyle of the elbow, caused by abnormalities in the wrist extensor muscles. There is debate as to whether there is an inflammatory component to this condition, thus some clinicians prefer the term lateral epicondylalgia. Different interventions exist for this condition, including physical therapy/stretching, braces, CSI, and rarely surgery. This article focuses on the utility of CSI.

Corticosteroid Injection for Lateral Epicondylalgia Syndrome: Efficacy

Many of the studies in the literature are poor in quality, but there have been some reasonably well-designed placebo-controlled studies from which some conclusions can be drawn.

A 2002 study by Smidt and colleagues[19] randomized 185 patients to 1 of 3 groups: CSI, physiotherapy, or wait and see (no treatment). There was no placebo injection group, but the therapist who rated the patients' symptoms was blinded to the treatment allocation. At the 6-week mark, the injection group had significantly higher success rates than the other two groups: 92% success versus 47% in the physiotherapy group and 32% in the no-treatment group. However, at 1 year the injection group had only a 69% success rate, compared with 92% for the physiotherapy group and 83% for the wait-and-see group. These differences were statistically significant.

A more recent study by Coombes and colleagues[20] found similar results. They randomized 165 patients in double-blind fashion to CSI or placebo injection, and the two groups were further randomized to physical therapy and bracing or no other treatment. Similar to other studies, at 4 weeks the CSI group was superior to the placebo group in pain relief, but only in the 2 groups that did not have the physical therapy and bracing intervention. The 2 injection groups were no different if the patients also had physical therapy and bracing. At 6 and 12 months, there were inferior results for the groups that had CSIs. For example, at 1 year the placebo injection groups had 96% complete or high-level improvement, compared with 83% in the CSI group. Similarly, at 1 year, the CSI group was much more likely to have a recurrence of the symptoms: 54% versus 12%. This percentage translated into a number needed to harm of 3, in terms of recurrent symptoms.

Corticosteroid Injection for Lateral Epicondylalgia Syndrome: Safety

The only side effects were local skin depigmentation and subcutaneous atrophy, which occurred in about 4% of the CS group and none of the placebo injection group. These changes were mild or moderate and self-limited.

Corticosteroid Injection for Lateral Epicondylalgia Syndrome: Cost

Total cost for CSI for epicondylalgia (medication and physician fee) can vary, but generally ranges from $50 to $200.

Corticosteroid Injection for Lateral Epicondylalgia Syndrome: Conclusions

CSIs for lateral epicondylalgia are equal to but not better than physical therapy at 4 weeks, but carry the longer-term harm of leading to higher recurrence rates and more symptoms at 6 and 12 months. Thus, CSIs for this syndrome should rarely be used, unless there is a compelling reason to offer the patient a short-term relief of symptoms in unusually severe cases.

GREATER TROCHANTERIC PAIN SYNDROME

Greater trochanteric pain syndrome (GTPS), previously termed trochanteric bursitis, is a condition characterized by pain in the lateral hip and thigh region, usually with palpable tenderness in the vicinity of the greater trochanter of the femur. The risk factors for this include obesity and knee osteoarthritis, among other situations that may change the normal biomechanics of gait. The exact pathophysiology is not known, but seems to involve problems in the trochanteric bursa as well as the gluteus medius, although inflammation has not definitively be shown to be involved in this disorder.[21] In many patients, the condition is chronic, and CSIs have been used for decades to treat GTPS, but most of the studies showing benefit to these injections have been methodologically flawed, such as failing to include a placebo group.[22–24]

Corticosteroid Injection for Treatment of Greater Trochanteric Pain Syndrome: Efficacy

Brinks and colleagues[25] randomized 120 patients with GTPS to CSI or usual care (oral analgesia, and physical therapy/exercises as desired by the patients). There was no placebo injection. At 3 months, more of the CSI group recovered compared with the usual-care group (55% versus 34%; NNT = 5). There was also a significant reduction in overall pain in the injection group. However, at 12 months 60% of patients in both groups had recovered, and there were no differences between the two groups in overall pain.

Rompe and colleagues[26] randomized 229 patients with refractory GTPS to 1 of 3 groups: home-training exercise program, a single local CSI, or repetitive low-energy shock wave treatment. At 1 month, the injection group had a much higher success rate (complete recovery or much improvement, 75% vs 7% for the home-training program and 13% for the shock wave therapy). However, at 6 months there was no difference between the CSI group and home-training group (51% and 41% success rates respectively), and at 15 months the shock wave and home-training groups were significantly more successful than the CSI group (80% success for home training vs 48% for the injection group). There were no significant side effects noted in this study.

Corticosteroid Injection for Treatment of Greater Trochanteric Pain Syndrome: Safety

Other than the aforementioned potential worse long-term outcomes, the studies do not report any significant negative consequences to CSI.

Corticosteroid Injection for Treatment of Greater Trochanteric Pain Syndrome: Cost

Total cost for CSI for GTPS (medication and physician fee) can vary, but generally ranges from $50 to $200.

Corticosteroid Injection for Treatment of Greater Trochanteric Pain Syndrome: Conclusion

CSI for treatment of GTPS is probably helpful in the short term, but possibly harmful in the long term (although only in 1 small study). In patients with significant pain, it is reasonable to do CSI for relief of symptoms, in concert with a physical therapy regimen.

DE QUERVAIN TENOSYNOVITIS

De Quervain tenosynovitis, or radial tenosynovitis, is characterized by pain at the thumb side of the wrist, caused by impairment of movement of 2 thumb tendons, the abductor pollicis longus and extensor pollicis brevis. It is often an overuse injury. CSIs have been used to treat this condition, although the studies showing benefit are few.

Corticosteroid Injection for De Quervain Tenosynovitis: Efficacy

In one study,[27] 18 pregnant or lactating women were randomized to CS plus bupivacaine injection or thumb spica splinting. After 6 days, all 9 of the women who had the injection were pain free, whereas none of the splinting group were pain free. No longer-term information was given from this study.

In another study,[28] 21 patients with de Quervain tenosynovitis were randomized to CS or saline injection. At 1 to 2 weeks of follow-up, 75% of the CS group had substantial improvement, compared with only 25% of the placebo group. The steroid responders were then followed for a year, and most, but not all, had maintenance of the improvement. The placebo group had a follow-up CSI as well, so no comparison at 1 year was possible between the two groups.

De Quervain Tenosynovitis: Safety

There were no significant side effects reported in these studies, but no long-term results are available. It is reasonable to assume that there are small potential risks such as tendon rupture and subcutaneous atrophy at the site, which have been reported occasionally.

De Quervain Tenosynovitis: Cost

Total cost for CSI for de Quervain tenosynovitis (medication and physician fee) can vary, but generally ranges from $50 to $200.

De Quervain Tenosynovitis: Conclusion

CSIs for de Quervain tenosynovitis are very helpful, and often curative, in the short term. There is no information to guide clinicians on long-term benefits or risks, but given the significant amount of pain many patients have with this condition it is reasonable to use CSI for primary treatment in patients who understand that there are no long-term data. For patients with lesser amounts of pain, it is reasonable to hold off on CSI and do splinting or other similar interventions.

DISEASES OF THE LUMBAR SPINE

There are different conditions that can affect the lumbar spine, and they differ in symptoms and pathophysiology, although they are related in some ways to degenerative arthritis, disc disease, or both. Sciatica, or lumbar radiculopathy, is a common condition that has a lifetime prevalence of about 4%.[29] It is characterized by radiating lower extremity pain below the knee, with or without low back pain, and is often accompanied by sensory neuropathic symptoms in a dermatomal distribution. Although the prognosis of sciatica is considered favorable, about 30% of patients have persistent symptoms at 1 year, and 5% to 10% proceed to surgery.[30] Similarly, lumbar spinal stenosis is a common condition affecting about 3% of patients, mostly older adults, and is caused by spinal canal narrowing by degenerative changes and congenital causes. This condition is characterized by bilateral radiating symptoms into the legs, and can lead to substantial debilitation. In addition, chronic low back pain is a very common condition that also leads to disability and loss of function.

Treatment of all of these conditions with physical therapy and oral analgesia has significant limitations, and surgery is considered a last resort in most cases. Thus, CSI into the lumbar spine region has emerged as an option in the treatment, and in Medicare recipients alone was used 1.5 million times in 2004,[31] and doubled in number between 1996 and 2007.[32] However, many of the studies have serious methodological flaws and the efficacy of this expensive intervention has been called into question.

Treatment of Lumbar Spine Disease with Corticosteroid Injection: Efficacy

In the WEST study,[32] 228 patients with unilateral sciatica for 1 to 18 months were randomized to 3 epidural injections of CS (triamcinolone) or saline (placebo group). At the 3 weeks, there was a small statistically significant benefit seen in the CSI group, in that 12% of them had greater than 75% improvement in symptoms, compared with 4% of the placebo injection group. Another way of looking at that is that almost all of the patients did not derive a large benefit. There was also a small improvement in overall function in the CS group. However, the benefits seen at 3 weeks disappeared at all time points between 6 weeks and 52 weeks, and the CSIs did not hasten the return to work over time or reduce overall analgesia use. In addition, the two groups did not differ in eventual surgical intervention (15% in both groups).

Another study assessed the utility of epidural CSIs in the treatment of lumbar spinal stenosis.[33] Four-hundred patients with moderate to severe pain thought to be from lumbar spinal stenosis were randomized to epidural injection of CS/lidocaine or lidocaine alone, with a second injection given at 3 weeks at the discretion of the physician. At 6 weeks, there was no significant difference between the two groups, with 38% reporting more than 50% improvement in leg pain and 20% having greater than 50% improvement in disability scores. Both groups had few side effects, with 2% experiencing headache after the procedure, and 3% reporting severe pain from the procedure. Note that 10% of the CS group had adrenal function suppression, compared with none in the lidocaine-alone group, as measured by morning cortisol values. The clinical relevance of this finding is debatable.

Two systematic review and meta-analysis articles were published in the past 4 years, concerning the efficacy of epidural CSIs for radiculopathy and spinal stenosis.[34,35] They similarly concluded, based on about 24 articles each, that epidural CSIs have short-term (a few weeks) benefit in the treatment of radiculopathy/sciatica but not spinal stenosis, and that these benefits are small and of debatable clinical relevance. They also determined that epidural CSIs have no significant benefit on pain relief or disability in the long term, and do not reduce the need for surgical intervention. Both reviews noted that many of the studies did not report harms, but those that did failed to show any substantial harm other than localized discomfort from the procedures themselves.

In addition, a review for the Cochrane group studied the efficacy of CSI for low back pain.[36,37] It concluded that the literature was heterogeneous, because of different locations of CSI (eg, facet joint, epidural, transforaminal), and there was insufficient evidence supporting the use of CSIs for chronic low back pain. The investigators did not rule out a possible benefit for certain subgroups, despite the lack of any solid evidence in support of this.

Treatment of Lumbar Spine Disease with Corticosteroid Injection: Safety

Various short-term mild side effects are reported, such as headache, nausea, and rash, all occurring in 1% to 3% of patients.[33] More serious complications such as dural puncture and infection are rare. Concerns have been raised about an increased risk of future vertebral fracture associated with repeated epidural CSI,[38] but this has not been definitively determined to be a real association. In addition, a much-publicized outbreak of aspergillus meningitis seriously sickened dozens of people and was fatal in several cases. This outbreak was traced back to 1 compounding pharmacy and contaminated methylprednisolone vials.[39]

Treatment of Lumbar Spine Disease with Corticosteroid Injection: Cost

The cost of CSI for lumbar spine disease can vary greatly and depends on the type of procedure used, the use of fluoroscopy, and the use of sedation. With all of these variables, costs can be as high as $2000 to $3000, especially if patients undergo repeat injections over time.

Treatment of Lumbar Spine Disease with Corticosteroid Injection: Conclusions

Epidural CSIs for the treatment of lumbar radiculopathy syndromes and spinal stenosis offer small short-term benefits (weeks) in some patients, but do not show long-term benefits or reduce the need for spinal surgery. The benefits are even more dubious in patients with chronic back pain who undergo facet joint or transforaminal CSI. As such, these interventions should be offered to patients only when a few weeks of pain relief is thought to be worth the cost of the intervention.

REFERENCES

1. Goroll AH, Mulley AG. Primary Care Medicine: Office Evaluation and Management of the Adult Patient. 4th edition. p. 860.
2. Arroll B, Goodyear-Smith F. Corticosteroid injections for osteoarthritis of the knee: meta-analysis. BMJ 2004;1136:1–5.
3. Hepper CT, Halvorson JJ, Duncan ST, et al. The efficacy and duration of intra-articular corticosteroid injection for knee osteoarthritis: a systematic review of level I studies. J Am Acad Orthop Surg 2009;17:638–46.
4. Bannuru R, Schmid C, Kent DM, et al. Comparative effectiveness of pharmacologic interventions in knee osteoarthritis: a systematic review and network meta-analysis. Ann Intern Med 2015;162(1):46–54.
5. Raynauld JP, Buckland-Wright C, Ward R, et al. Safety and efficacy of long-term intraarticular steroid injections in osteoarthritis of the knee: a randomized, double-blind, placebo-controlled trial. Arthritis Rheum 2003 Feb;48(2):370–7.
6. Juni P, Hari R, Rutjes AW, et al. Intra-articular corticosteroids for knee osteoarthritis. Cochrane Database Syst Rev 2015;(10):CD005328.
7. Hochberg M, Altman R, April KT, et al. American College of Rheumatology 2012 recommendations for the use of nonpharmacologic and pharmacologic therapies in osteoarthritis of the hand, hip, and knee. Arthritis Care Res (Hoboken) 2012; 64(4):465–74.

8. Jevsevar DS. Treatment of osteoarthritis of the knee: evidence-based guideline, 2nd edition. J Am Acad Orthop Surg 2013;21:571. American Academy of Orthopedic Surgery. Treatment of Osteoarthritis of the Knee, second edition. Summary of Recommendations. Available at: AAOS.org. Accessed March 1, 2016.

9. Bragantini A, Cassini M, De B, et al. Controlled single-blind trial of intra-articularly injected hyaluronic acid (Hyalgan®) in osteoarthritis of the knee. Clin Trials J 1987;24:333–40.

10. Arrich J, Piribauer F, Mad P, et al. Intra-articular hyaluronic acid for the treatment of osteoarthritis of the knee: systematic review and meta-analysis. CMAJ 2005; 172(8):1039–43.

11. Rutjes A, Anne WS, Juni P, et al. Viscosupplementation for osteoarthritis of the knee: a systematic review and meta-analysis. Ann Intern Med 2012;157(3): 180–91.

12. Bellamy N, Campbell J, Robinson V, et al. Intraarticular corticosteroid for treatment of osteoarthritis of the knee. Cochrane Database Syst Rev 2006.

13. Koester M, Dunn W, Kuhn J, et al. The efficacy of subacromial corticosteroid injection in the treatment of rotator cuff disease: a systematic review. J Am Acad Orthop Surg 2007;15:3–11.

14. Arroll B, Goodyear-Smith F. Corticosteroid injections for the painful shoulder: a meta-analysis. Br J Gen Pract 2005;55:224–8.

15. Alvarez C, Litchfield R, Jackowski D, et al. A prospective double-blind randomized clinical trial comparing subacromial injection of betamethasone and xylocaine to xylocaine alone in chronic rotator cuff tendinosis. Am J Sports Med 2005;33(2):255–62.

16. Rhon D, Boyles R, Cleland J. One-year outcome of subacromial corticosteroid injection compared with manual physical therapy for the management of the unilateral shoulder impingement syndrome. Ann Intern Med 2014;161:161–9.

17. Drezner JA, Sennett BJ. Subacromial septic bursitis associated with isotretinoin therapy and corticosteroid injection. J Am Board Fam Pract 2004;17: 299–302.

18. Watson M. Major ruptures of the rotator cuff. The results of surgical repair in 89 patients. J Bone Joint Surg Br 1985;67:618–24.

19. Smidt N, van der Windt DA, Assendelft WJ, et al. Corticosteroid injections, physiotherapy, or a wait-and-see policy for lateral epicondylitis: a randomised controlled trial. Lancet 2002;359(9307):657–62.

20. Coombes BK, Bisset L, Brooks P, et al. Effect of corticosteroid injection, physiotherapy, or both on clinical outcomes in patients with unilateral lateral epicondylalgia: a randomized controlled trial. JAMA 2013;309(5):461–9.

21. Silva F, Adams T, Feinstein J, et al. Trochanteric bursitis: refuting the myth of inflammation. J Clin Rheumatol 2008;14(2):82–6.

22. Bird PA, Oakley SP, Shnier R, et al. Prospective evaluation of magnetic resonance imaging and physical examination findings in patients with greater trochanteric pain syndrome. Arthritis Rheum 2001;44(9):2138–45.

23. Lievense A, Bierma-Zeinstra S, Schouten B, et al. Prognosis of trochanteric pain in primary care. Br J Gen Pract 2005;55(512):199–204.

24. Shbeeb MI, O'Duffy JD, Michet CJ, et al. Evaluation of glucocorticoid injection for the treatment of trochanteric bursitis. J Rheumatol 1996;23(12):2104–6.

25. Brink A, Van Rijn R, Willemsen S, et al. Corticosteroid injections for greater trochanteric pain syndrome: a randomized controlled trial in primary care. Ann Fam Med 2011;9:226–34.

26. Rompe JD, Segal NA, Cacchio A, et al. Home training, local corticosteroid injection, or radial shock wave therapy for greater trochanter pain syndrome. Am J Sports Med 2009;37(10):1981–90.

27. Avci S, Yilmaz C, Sayli U. Comparison of nonsurgical treatment measures of De Quervain's disease of pregnancy and lactation. J Hand Surg 2002;37A(2): 322–4.

28. Peters-Veluthamaningal C, Winters JC, Groenier KH, et al. Randomised controlled trial of local corticosteroid injections for de Quervain's tenosynovitis in general practice. BMC Musculoskelet Disord 2009;10:131–6.

29. Heliovaara M, impivaara O, Sievers K, et al. Lumbar disc syndrome in Finland. J Epidemiol Community Health 1987;41:251–8.

30. Bush K, Cowan N, Katz DE, et al. The natural history of sciatica associated with disc pathology: a prospective study with clinical and independent radiological follow-up. Spine (Phila Pa 1976) 1992;17(10):1205–12.

31. Manchikanti I. Medicare in interventional pain management: a critical analysis. Pain Physician 2006;9:171–97.

32. Manchikanti L, Pampati V, Boswell MV, et al. Analysis of the growth of epidural injections and costs in the Medicare population: a comparative evaluation of 1997, 2002, and 2006 data. Pain Physician 2010;13(3):199–212.

33. Arden NK, Price C, Reading I, et al. A multicenter randomized controlled trial of epidural corticosteroid injections for sciatica: the WEST study. Rheumatology 2005;44:1399–406.

34. Friedly J, Comstok B, Turner JA, et al. A randomized trial of epidural steroid injections for spinal stenosis. N Engl J Med 2014;371:11–21.

35. Pinto RZ, Maher CG, Ferreira ML, et al. Epidural corticosteroid injections in the management of sciatica. Ann Intern Med 2012;57:865–77.

36. Chou R, Hashimoto R, Friedly J, et al. Epidural corticosteroid injections for radiculopathy and spinal stenosis. Ann Intern Med 2015;163:373–81.

37. Staal JB, de Bie R, de Vet HC, et al. Injection therapy for subacute and chronic low-back pain. Cochrane Database Syst Rev 2008;(3):CD001824.

38. Mandel S, Schilling J, Peterson E, et al. A retrospective analysis of vertebral body fractures following epidural steroid injections. J Bone Joint Surg Am 2013;95: 961–4.

39. Centers for Disease Control and Prevention (CDC). Multistate outbreak of fungal infection associated with injection of methylprednisolone acetate solution from a single compounding pharmacy - United States, 2012. MMWR Morb Mortal Wkly Rep 2012;61:839.

Utilization and Safety of Common Over-the-Counter Dietary/Nutritional Supplements, Herbal Agents, and Homeopathic Compounds for Disease Prevention

(®) CrossMark

Ruchir Trivedi, MD, MMedSci, MRCP(UK)[a],*,
Marissa C. Salvo, PharmD, BCACP[b]

KEYWORDS

- Dietary supplement • Over-the-counter (OTC) supplements • Herbal
- Micronutrients • Homeopathic compound • Drug interactions
- Regulation of dietary supplements

KEY POINTS

- Available evidence supporting the use of dietary supplements varies based on the supplement and the indication for which it is being used.
- This review highlights several disease states and the available evidence regarding dietary supplement use.
- Manufacturers, rather than the US Food and Drug Administration, are responsible for evaluating the safety and labeling of dietary supplements before marketing.
- Clinicians need to remain abreast of emerging evidence and recommendations regarding the use of dietary supplements.

INTRODUCTION

The Dietary Supplement Health and Education Act of 1994 (DSHEA) classifies dietary supplements as vitamins, minerals, herbs or other botanicals, and amino acids intended to supplement diet.[1] Manufacturers are responsible for evaluating the safety and labeling of their products before marketing to ensure it meets DSHEA

Disclosure Statement: The authors have nothing to disclose.
[a] Division of Nephrology, Department of Medicine, University of Connecticut School of Medicine, 263 Farmington Avenue, Farmington, CT 06032, USA; [b] Department of Pharmacy Practice, University of Connecticut School of Pharmacy, 69 North Eagleville Road, Unit 3092, Storrs, CT 06269, USA
* Corresponding author.
E-mail address: Rtrivedi@uchc.edu

Med Clin N Am 100 (2016) 1089–1099
http://dx.doi.org/10.1016/j.mcna.2016.04.017
0025-7125/16/$ – see front matter © 2016 Elsevier Inc. All rights reserved.

regulations.[2,3] Recent data suggest almost one-third of US children and adults use health supplements.[4,5] Given that there are more than 55,000 supplements and micronutrients, a detailed assessment of preventive efficacy of all available products is beyond scope of this review. This article reviews available evidence for dietary supplements in select disease categories. Readers are referred to the Natural Medicine comprehensive database (http://www.naturaldatabase.com) and the Cochrane database for in-depth reviews.

DISEASES OF ALLERGY AND IMMUNOLOGY

Over the past 20 years, the prevalence of allergies in industrialized countries has increased 5-fold, from approximately 4% to an estimated 20%.[6] Allergic diseases include food allergies, atopic dermatitis (eczema), asthma, and allergic rhinitis (hay fever). There is growing evidence that rising propensity for allergy and inflammation may be programmed in very early life. This evidence has led to widespread use of complementary therapies with the expectation for improvement in childhood atopy and asthma.[7]

Fish oils are major sources of omega-3 long chain fatty acids (ω-3 fatty acids). ω-3 fatty acids can reduce plasma triacylglycerols (triglycerides) and increase high-density lipoprotein cholesterol. Fish oils have also been shown to lower blood pressure and improve vascular reactivity.[8] Dietary reduction in ω-3 fatty acid intake over the last 20 to 30 years coincides with a dramatic increase in the incidence of asthma and allergic diseases. Antiinflammatory properties of ω-3 fatty acids can inhibit allergic inflammatory and immunoglobulin E (IgE)-mediated immune responses, especially when given early, before the establishment of allergic immune response in vitro. This plausible mechanism resulted in widespread use of ω-3 supplementation in pregnancy with the aim to reduce neonatal allergic diseases. However, maternal supplementation of ω-3 fatty acids failed to show a decline in incidence of IgE-mediated allergic rhinitis or IgE-mediated asthma.[8,9]

Throughout evolution, microbial genes and metabolites have become an integral part of human physiology, metabolism, and immune responses. Rapid urbanization, widespread antibiotics use, commercial agricultural practices, environmental pollutants, highly processed foods/beverages, and socioeconomic disparities are all implicated in compromising a vast and individually distinct residential microbial community in humans, collectively known as human microbiome. Alteration of the human microbiome and decline in intestinal biodiversity may result in defective or inadequate immune responses.[10] Early observations suggest that reduced intestinal biodiversity may be a fundamental factor in rising propensity of allergic and some inflammatory diseases. The use of mixed strain probiotics (eg, combination of lactobacilli, bifidobacteria, and other probiotic organisms) has been explored with an aim to repopulate intestinal microbial biodiversity.[7,10,11] A review of studies that used rigorous methodologies do seem to indicate that maternal probiotic use may decrease the incidence of eczema in high-risk infants.[7] Similar benefits, however, were not shown with other allergic conditions. Hence, the recommendation to use probiotics for atopic conditions should be very restrictive.

The use of vitamin C, bitter orange, ephedra, and grape seed extracts for allergic rhinitis are probably ineffective and may even be harmful. Bitter orange and ephedra are used as dietary supplements and as appetite suppressants to achieve weight loss. Both of these compounds have significant side-effect profiles that include worsening hypertension and severe vasoconstriction that may result in intestinal angina or coronary ischemia. Grape seed extract contains antioxidants, which can help prevent damage caused by highly reactive free radicals that damage cell function and promote inflammation. The side-effect profile is low but includes nausea, dry itchy scalp, headaches, and high blood pressure in some patients. Studies demonstrating efficacy are equivocal.[12] It is important to counsel patients that Echinacea (American coneflower), feverfew (also used in migraine), and chamomile (also used in infantile colic, mouth ulcers, and anxiety disorders) are members of the ragweed family and could enhance allergic reactions. Echinacea is used for its immune stimulant property to "fight colds" and help mount robust immune responses. Study results are mixed on whether echinacea can prevent or effectively treat upper respiratory tract infections such as the common cold or help allergic responses.[10] Individuals with asthma or atopy (a genetic tendency toward allergic reactions) are more likely to have an allergic reaction when taking echinacea; hence, unmonitored use should be discouraged. Feverfew and chamomile are not well studied; hence, there is little evidence to support its use at present.[10]

UROLOGICAL DISEASES: BENIGN PROSTATIC HYPERPLASIA AND URINARY TRACT INFECTION

Saw palmetto, which seems to have antiandrogenic, antiproliferative, and anti-inflammatory properties, is the best known and most widely used supplement for benign prostatic hyperplasia (BPH). It has a 5-α reductase inhibitory effect, which is similar to but far less potent than prescription medications, such as finasteride. Saw palmetto, in theory, may reduce prostate growth by preventing the conversion of testosterone to dihydrotestosterone.[11,12] However, a study in 369 older men demonstrated that saw palmetto extract administered at up to 3 times the standard daily dose (320 mg) did not reduce the urinary symptoms associated with BPH more than placebo.[11]

Pygeum (also known as African plum tree) and β-sitosterol have been studied for treating BPH-related symptoms, and they appear to decrease nocturia, increase urine flow, and decrease residual urine volume. Pygeum extract contains a 5-lipoxygenase metabolite that may contribute to its anti-inflammatory effects. Antiproliferative and apoptotic effects of pygeum on prostate fibroblasts and myofibroblasts are due to downregulation of transforming growth factor B1 (TGFB1) and inhibition of fibroblast growth factor 2.[11] β-Sitosterol downregulates TGFB1 and reduces absorption of cholesterol.[12] β-Sitosterol's use may be a viable option for men who have BPH and hypercholesterolemia.[12] Garlic, selenium, and zinc are sometimes used; however, data supporting their efficacy are sparse.

Cranberry is used for both chronic, nonbacterial prostatitis and urinary tract infection (UTI) prevention. Dried cranberry 500 mg 3 times daily for 6 months may improve lower urinary symptoms (such as frequency, urgency, and hesitancy) and reduces prostate-specific antigen (PSA) levels in men more than 45 years of age with elevated PSA levels, a negative prostate biopsy, and clinically confirmed nonbacterial prostatitis.[13] Cranberry primarily works to decrease the binding and invasion of *Escherichia coli* and pseudomonas to the uroepithelial cell. One systematic review found only weak evidence for its use in women with recurrent UTI.[14] Patients with neurogenic bladder or requiring clean intermittent catheterization did not show significant benefits.[14] Unfortunately, efficacy of cranberry extract is not reproducible, at best mild; hence, its widespread use cannot be advocated.[14]

BONE HEALTH

Calcium intake of less than 800 mg per day is associated with bone mineral density (BMD) loss in postmenopausal and perimenopausal women. Increasing intake to 1200 mg per day, along with increased physical activity, can decrease age associated

BMD loss.[15] Supplemental calcium is most beneficial when baseline calcium intake is low.

For osteoporosis prevention, calcium (1000–1200 mg) should be taken daily with vitamin D (800–1000 International Units).[2,15] Available evidence to support use of calcium in hip fracture prevention is limited to patients with severe vitamin D deficiency.[16] Any potential benefits of high doses of calcium (>2000 mg/d) must be weighed against its gastrointestinal (GI) side effects, potential increase in incidence of renal calculi, and possible increase in non-ST elevation myocardial infarction.[16,17] Deposition of calcium into arterial walls is an integral part of the atherosclerotic process; therefore, excessive and/or unsupervised calcium supplementation may increase adverse cardiovascular outcomes, especially in patients with end-stage chronic kidney disease. Higher than recommended doses of vitamin D should be discouraged for its potential harm in absence of strong outcome data.[17]

Chromium, copper, dehydroepiandrosterone (DHEA), evening primrose oil, red clover, black cohosh, chondroitin sulfate, and shark cartilage are other dietary supplements marketed for their presumed bone health benefits. Human evidence is sparse to nonexistent; therefore, their use is not recommended.

VIRAL UPPER RESPIRATORY TRACT INFECTIONS AND INFLUENZA (COLDS AND FLU)

Commonly marketed products such as echinacea, vitamin C, and zinc to provide "immune support" do not seem to be effective in the prevention of "colds" in adults. Zinc at doses 10 to 15 mg daily has been shown to decrease the number of colds per year in children, antibiotic usage, and absent school days (number needed to treat: 6) in 2 randomized control trials.[18] However, these studies have some methodological concerns. Although there are no biological reasons to suggest that adults would not benefit from zinc therapy, direct evidence showing similar reduction in the number of colds per year is lacking.

Panax ginseng, also known as Asian ginseng, may protect against colds and improve response to the influenza vaccine.[19] Approximately 40 different ginsenosides are identified, and they appear to be responsible for properties such as vasorelaxation, antioxidation, anti-inflammation, and anticancer.[19] Ginsenosides can inhibit reactive oxygen species production, stimulate nitric oxide production, increase immune function via stimulating cell-mediated immunity, improve glucose metabolism, enhance central nervous system function, and prevent cardiovascular or other diseases.[19,20] Type 2 diabetes mellitus (DM) and chronic respiratory failure are 2 emerging indications that merit further study of panax ginseng.[18]

CARDIOVASCULAR DISEASE

Cardiovascular disease (CVD) is the leading global cause of death, accounting for an estimated 17.3 million deaths per year, with an expected growth to more than 23 million by 2030.[21] Despite the paucity of hard clinical data, dietary supplement use is widespread for cardiovascular health. Garlic, due to an organosulfur compound allicin, is believed to have a lipid-lowering effect.[22] However, overall data suggest considerable inconsistencies and variable results in lowering of total cholesterol and low-density lipoprotein (LDL).[22]

Green tea is a rich source of flavonoids and compounds commonly known as "green tea catechins." Animal studies have shown that green tea catechins reduce intestinal cholesterol absorption, reduce hepatic cholesterol content, and cause upregulation of LDL-receptors with increased activity.[23] The Ohsaki study—a population-based, prospective cohort study of 40,530 Japanese adults with almost 11 years of follow-up—showed that the consumption of green tea was inversely associated with cardiovascular and all-cause mortality.[23] The true effect of green tea extract on human cardiovascular health is difficult to ascertain because most positive studies have a small sample size and variable improvement in lipid profile.

Guggul and red yeast rice are widely used with the expectation to improve lipid profile and plaque stability.[24] Red yeast extract, during fermentation, can produce 14 different monacolins with hydroxymethylglutaryl-coenzyme A (HMG-CoA) reductase inhibitor activity, explaining the popularity of red yeast rice as a replacement to statin therapy, especially in statin-intolerant patients.[22] A major limitation to the widespread recommendation of red yeast rice is its variability in extract and quantity per dose.[22,24]

ω-3 fatty acids may enhance vasodilatation by stimulating nitric oxide and vasodilatory prostaglandins and can cause suppression of the renin-angiotensin-aldosterone system.[25] ω-3 fatty acid consumption has been associated with reduced risk of cardiac mortality, by means of membrane stabilization, inhibition of platelet aggregation, favorable modifications of the lipid profile, and a decrease in blood pressure, and a reduction of the inflammatory response of the endothelium.[26] ω-3 fatty acid supplementation is a subject of intense research over many years because of multiple potential benefits; however, a recent meta-analysis failed to show improvement in hard clinical outcomes such as myocardial infarction, sudden cardiac death, stroke, or all-cause mortality.[27]

In addition to its lipid-lowering and blood pressure–lowering effects, ω-3 fatty acids and fish oil supplementation have been used in a variety of disorders including IgA nephropathy, prevention of clotting with arteriovenous graft for dialysis, generalized systemic inflammation, and cancer prevention. In order to derive clinically measurable benefit, large doses need to be taken. Unfortunately, stringent clinical trial data with existing gold standards for individual conditions are not available. Potential contaminants of ω-3 fatty acids include mercury, dioxins, and polychlorinated biphenyls. Other supplements often used to support cardiovascular health include vitamin E, flavonoids, and coenzyme Q10 (CoQ10). The HOPE trial, a definitive clinical trial relating vitamin E supplementation to cardiovascular outcomes, revealed no effect on the incidence of myocardial infarction, stroke, or death.[28,29] Flavonoids, which are polyphenolic antioxidants, are found in a variety of foods such as tea, onions, apples, and dark chocolates. Overzealous approximation and estimates from small short-term studies are sometimes used to highlight long-term benefits of dark chocolate. One such estimate suggests that eating 50 g of dark chocolate per day may reduce one's risk of CVD by 10.5% (95% confidence interval 7.0%–13.5%).[25,28]

CoQ10 is an essential mitochondrial cofactor and free radical scavenger with possible beneficial effects in patients with cardiomyopathy, postcardiac arrest, septic shock, and neurodegenerative disorders.[29] CoQ10, located within the inner mitochondrial membrane, acts as an electron transport mediator and is often used with the expectation to prevent statin-induced myopathy.[29] Statins block farnesyl pyrophosphate, an intermediate for CoQ10 synthesis, and decrease HMG-CoA reductase activity, which plays a role in CoQ10 biosynthesis. Although CoQ10 administration increases plasma CoQ10,[24] there is insufficient evidence that supplementation has consistent clinical benefit in reducing statin-related myopathy. Adverse effects are few and seem to be limited to GI intolerance in small studies.[28]

DEPRESSION

Depression has been identified as one of the most common indication to use complementary and alternative medicine.

St. John's wort is the best known natural antidepressant. It inhibits the reuptake of serotonin, norepinephrine, and dopamine. Hypericin was thought to be the major constituent in St. John's wort; however, more recent studies suggest hyperforin and hyperforin-like substances are the active ingredients.[30,31] Most of the evidence shows that St. John's wort is effective for improving mood and reducing insomnia and somatic symptoms of depression in patients with mild to moderate depression.[31] Although St. John's wort is considered to be comparable in efficacy to low-dose tricyclic antidepressants and selective serotonin reuptake inhibitors,[32] randomized clinical trial data consider St. John's wort no better than placebo.[30]

St. John's wort is an inducer of the cytochrome (CYP) P-450 liver enzyme system, specifically CYP3A4, leading to altered metabolism of many pharmaceuticals coadministered with the wort.[30] Patients should be informed that even though St. John's wort is likely to be effective, it is not necessarily the best choice for therapy. There is no reliable evidence that St. John's wort is better tolerated than conventional antidepressants,[41] and there is potential for significant drug interactions. Serotonin syndrome can occur when St. John's wort is taken alone or when it is combined with other drugs that increase serotonin levels. Hypertensive crisis has also been reported in patients taking St. John's wort and eating tyramine-containing food (aged cheeses, smoked fish, and so on) or drinking red wine (**Table 1**).

DIABETES MELLITUS

Survey data suggest that up to 30% to 70% of patients with DM use some form of alternative medicine over the course of a year.[33] Banaba leaf extract, bitter melon, fenugreek, gymnema, and ivy gourd are touted to have insulinlike activity and can also activate insulin receptors. Bitter melon can potentiate the hypoglycemic effect of antidiabetic medications.[34] The antidiabetic effect of fenugreek seeds may be secondary to its effect on slowing GI absorption of carbohydrates and increasing insulin release. Patients taking antiplatelet agents should be closely monitored because Fenugreek may enhance their antiplatelet activity and increase bleeding risks.[34,35]

Cinnamon, chromium, magnesium, panax ginseng, prickly pear cactus, soy, and vanadium are also increasingly being used for their effect as insulin sensitizers.[34,35] Cinnamon contains coumarin constituents that have been linked to liver damage when taken in very high doses.[36] Cinnamon, when subjected to rigorous trials, failed to improve HbA1c in a clinically significant manner. Excessive chromium intake might cause renal injury and potentially worsen existing renal disease.

Magnesium is actively involved as a cofactor in carbohydrate metabolism and glycemic control.[37,38] Reduced dietary magnesium intake can serve as a risk factor

| Table 1 | |
Select drug interaction with St John's wort	
Antiepileptics such as phenytoin	Digoxin and theophylline
Antihistamines such as fexofenadine	Immunosuppressants, such as cyclosporine and tacrolimus
Imatinib	Antiretrovirals, such as indinavir
Selective serotonin reuptake inhibitors such as paroxitine	Statins, such as Simvastatin
Oral contraceptives	Migraine medications, such as sumatriptan
Antiplatelet and anticoagulants such as clopidogrel and warfarin	Benzodiazepines, such as alprazolam

for impaired glucose regulation.[38] There is some evidence that chronic magnesium supplementation may delay the progression from impaired glucose regulation to type 2 DM. The effects of oral magnesium supplementation as an adjunct therapy for established type 2 DM are quite heterogeneous and cannot be supported by high-quality evidence.[38]

OBESITY

Approximately one-third of the US population who are trying to lose weight use a dietary supplement.[39] St. John's wort, 5-hydroxytryptophan (5-HTP), and Hoodia (cactuslike stem succulent) are all known for their appetite-suppressant effects. St John's wort has some appetite-suppressant activity. Serotonin syndrome and other drug interactions can be life threatening with St. John's wort (see **Table 1**). Although 5-HTP can cause a decreased intake of carbohydrates by causing early satiety, potential side effects such as serotonin syndrome and eosinophilia myalgia syndrome mandate extreme caution, and it is best to avoid its use. Hoodia extract, commonly taken for its appetite-suppressant effects, when given to healthy volunteers for 2 weeks significantly increased blood pressure, heart rate, bilirubin, and alkaline phosphatase levels.[40]

Numerous dietary supplements are marketed for their thermogenic or "fat-burning "effect. Ephedra, bitter orange, and dimethylamylamine are available in various preworkout supplements to promote fat burning. Patients should be cautioned about their use given their cardiovascular side effects, including hypertension and tachyarrhythmias.

Starch absorption inhibitors blockers like Chitosan and bean pod (high fiber content) are also used widely. Raspberry ketone and green coffee extract are becoming more popular with the general public. Widespread use of any of these supplements cannot be supported due to lack of credible evidence.

INTERACTION OF NUTRITIONAL SUPPLEMENTS WITH PRESCRIPTION MEDICATIONS

Widespread use of dietary supplements with little regulation raises safety concerns. In the United States, annually, an estimated 23,000 emergency department (ER) visits and 2000 hospitalizations are attributed to adverse events related to dietary supplements.[41] More than 25% of these visits involve individuals between 20 and 34 years of age, often a healthy population.[43] Weight loss and energy products are responsible for more than 50% of all visits, and the most common symptoms are cardiovascular in nature.

The potential for dietary supplement and prescription drug interactions remains an area of significant concern. One such drug interaction is the CYP enzyme system and St. John's wort. The CYP 3A4 enzyme is involved in the metabolism of more than 50% of all drugs. Therefore, supplements such as St. John's wort, garlic, DHEA, and others that alter this enzyme system can interact with numerous prescription drugs. Unfortunately, there are no reliable estimates showing how often drug-supplement interactions occur or how severe these interactions are in patients at risk and in the population in general. Moreover, the US Food and Drug Administration (FDA) necessitates reporting the shape and size of prescription medications (<22 nm); however, these requirements do not apply to supplements. Consequently, among older adults, approximately 40% of dietary supplement–related adverse reactions requiring ER visits were due to swallowing problems.[41]

Table 2 provides a short list of common drug-supplement interactions.

Table 2
Select dietary supplement-prescription drug interactions

Dietary Supplement-Prescription Drug Interactions	Significant Clinical Effects
Grapefruit: Selectively *inhibit* gut CYP3A4 up to 24 h (separating medications and grapefruit may not help)	Increased GI absorption of clindamycin, diltiazem, losartan, sitagliptin
St. John's wort: potent *inducer* of CYP3A4	Decrease effect of many drugs such as oral contraceptives, Imatinib, human immunodeficiency virus protease inhibitors, amitriptyline, digoxin, cyclosporine, tacrolimus, phenytoin, and statins Clopidogrel is a prodrug. It needs to be metabolized by CYP3A4 to become active, so taking it with St. John's wort *increases* clopidogrel effect (bleeding)
Calcium: binds to various antibiotics such as quinolone and tetracycline, antiepileptics such as phenytoin and phenobarbital, levothyroxine, and bisphosphonates	Calcium can bind and reduce absorption of some prescription medications like levothyroxine. To avoid this interaction, advise patients to take calcium supplements at least 4 h apart
Noni juice: increased risk of hyperkalemia with concomitant use of ACE inhibitors, angiotensin receptor blockers, aldosterone antagonists, and bactrim	Noni juice is high in potassium; combination therapy with other medications that increases potassium results in increased risk of hyperkalemia
Ginkgo: lower seizure threshold and increased bleeding risks	Avoid concomitant use with antiepileptics Avoid concomitant use with nonsteroidal anti-inflammatory agents, clopidogrel, and warfarin
Bitter orange: QT prolongation	Avoid coadministration with other medications that also prolong the QT interval, such as amiodarone, dofetilide ibutilide, procainamide, quinidine, sotalol, linezolid, and thioridazine

HOMEOPATHIC COMPOUNDS

A homeopathic compound has known effects that mimic the symptoms, syndrome, or condition that it is administered to treat and is manufactured in accordance with the Homeopathic Pharmacopoeia of the United States.[42,43] The phrase "let likes be cured by likes" is the underlying principle of homeopathic medicine, conveying the thought that disease symptoms can be cured by using small doses of homeopathic compounds (dilutions obtained from a variety of sources such as plants, minerals, or animals), which produce similar symptoms in healthy individuals.[43] Because homeopathic compounds are highly individualized with no standardized prescribing, the National Center for Complementary and Integrative Health states that there is little evidence supporting the use of homeopathy as effective treatment for any specific medical condition.[43]

SUMMARY

Available evidence supporting the use of dietary supplements varies based on the supplement and its use. Currently, dietary supplements available in the United States are neither standardized nor regulated. Standardization of dietary supplements to meet the testing and auditing criteria of the US Pharmacopeia (USP) is voluntary. A product that meets the criteria carries a "USP Verified Mark" on its label. Patients should be encouraged to look for this label for confidence in the ingredients listed on the label, knowledge that it is free of contaminants, and understanding that it is manufactured according to FDA and USP Good Manufacturing Practices in a sanitary and well-controlled process.[44] Clinicians need to remain abreast of emerging evidence and recommendations regarding the use of dietary supplements, their effectiveness in relationship to the cost burden to patients, and potential prescription drug-supplement interactions.

REFERENCES

1. Dietary Supplement Health and Education Act of 1994. Dietary Supplement Health and Education Act of 1994 1994;Public Law 103–417(108 stat 4325).
2. Bailey RL, West KP Jr, Black RE. The epidemiology of global micronutrient deficiencies. Ann Nutr Metab 2015;66:22–33.
3. Bailey RL, Gahche JJ, Thomas PR, et al. Why US children use dietary supplements. Pediatr Res 2013;74(6):737–41.
4. Wallace TC. Twenty years of the dietary supplement health and education act—how should dietary supplements be regulated? J Nutr 2015;145(8):1683–6.
5. Halila GC, Junior EH, Otuki MF, et al. The practice of OTC counseling by community pharmacists in Parana, Brazil. Pharmacy Practice 2015;13(4):597.
6. Pawanker R, Canonica GW, Holgate ST, et al, editors. WAO white book on allergy. World Allergy Organization (WAO); 2011.
7. Rueter K, Haynes A, Prescott SL. Developing primary intervention strategies to prevent allergic disease. Curr Allergy Asthma Rep 2015;15(7):40.
8. Barden AE, Dunstan JA, Beilin LJ, et al. n-3 fatty acid supplementation during pregnancy in women with allergic disease: effects on blood pressure, and maternal and fetal lipids. Clin Sci (Lond) 2006;111(4):289–94.
9. Vandenplas Y, Huys G, Daube G. Probiotics: an update. J Pediatr 2015;91(1):6–21.
10. Katz AE, Darves-Bornoz A. Complementary therapy. Anonymous; 2014. p. 154–63.
11. Cheetham PJ. Role of complimentary therapy for male LUTS. Curr Urol Rep 2013;14(6):606–13.
12. Signorello LB, Tzonou A, Lagiou P, et al. The epidemiology of benign prostatic hyperplasia: a study in Greece. BJU Int 1999;84(3):286–91.
13. Vidlar A, Vostalova J, Ulrichova J, et al. The effectiveness of dried cranberries (vaccinium macrocarpon) in men with lower urinary tract symptoms. Br J Nutr 2010;104(8):1181–9.
14. Jepson RG, Williams G, Craig JC. Cranberries for preventing urinary tract infections. Cochrane Database Syst Rev 2012;(10):CD001321.
15. Ströhle A, Hadji P, Hahn A. Calcium and bone health—goodbye, calcium supplements? Climacteric 2015;18(5):702–14.
16. Reid IR, Bristow SM, Bolland MJ. Calcium supplements: benefits and risks. J Intern Med 2015;278(4):354–68.
17. Bolland MJ, Avenell A, Baron JA, et al. Effect of calcium supplements on risk of myocardial infarction and cardiovascular events: meta-analysis. BMJ 2010;341(7767):289.
18. Allan GM, Arroll B. Prevention and treatment of the common cold: making sense of the evidence. CMAJ 2014;186(3):190–9.

19. Shergis JL, Zhang AL, Zhou W, et al. Panax ginseng in randomised controlled trials: a systematic review. Phytother Res 2013;27(7):949–65.
20. Shishtar E, Sievenpiper JL, Djedovic V, et al. The effect of ginseng (the genus panax) on glycemic control: a systematic review and meta-analysis of randomized controlled clinical trials. PLoS One 2014;9(9):e107391.
21. Ezzati M, Obermeyer Z, Tzoulaki I, et al. Contributions of risk factors and medical care to cardiovascular mortality trends. Nat Rev Cardiol 2015;12(9):508–30.
22. Danavi JV, Memon SB, Phan BAP. Statin alternatives: a review of over-the-counter lipid-lowering supplements. Altern Complement Ther 2015;21(5):198–209.
23. Kuriyama S, Shimazu T, Ohmori K, et al. Green tea consumption and mortality due to cardiovascular disease, cancer, and all causes in Japan: the Ohsaki Study. J Am Med Assoc 2006;296(10):1255–65.
24. Whayne TF Jr. What should medical practitioners know about the role of alternative medicines in cardiovascular disease management? Cardiovasc Ther 2010; 28(2):106–23.
25. Sirtori CR, Arnoldi A, Cicero AFG. Nutraceuticals for blood pressure control. Ann Med 2015;47(6):447–56.
26. Tur JA, Bibiloni MM, Sureda A, et al. Dietary sources of omega 3 fatty acids: public health risks and benefits. Br J Nutr 2012;107(Suppl 2):S23–52.
27. Katz DL. Lifestyle and dietary modification for prevention of heart failure. Med Clin North Am 2004;88(5):1295–320.
28. Reddy KS. Diet and cardiovascular disease. Anonymous; 2010. p. 304–27.
29. Cocchi MN, Giberson B, Berg K, et al. Coenzyme Q10 levels are low and associated with increased mortality in post-cardiac arrest patients. Resuscitation 2012;83(8):991–5.
30. Holstege CP, Mitchell K, Barlotta K, et al. Toxicity and drug interactions associated with herbal products: ephedra and St. John's wort. Med Clin North Am 2005;89(6):1225–57.
31. Dostalek M, Stark AK. St John's wort (Hypericum Perforatum L.). Anonymous; 2012. p. 583–610.
32. Szegedi A, Kohnen R, Dienel A, et al. Acute treatment of moderate to severe depression with hypericum extract WS 5570 (St John's wort): randomised controlled double blind non-inferiority trial versus paroxetine. BMJ 2005; 330(7490):503–6.
33. Nahin RL, Byrd-Clark D, Stussman BJ, et al. Disease severity is associated with the use of complementary medicine to treat or manage type-2 diabetes: data from the 2002 and 2007 National Health Interview Survey. BMC Complement Altern Med 2012;12:193.
34. Hosein Farzaei M, Rahimi R, Farzaei F, et al. Traditional medicinal herbs for the management of diabetes and its complications: an evidence-based review. Int J Pharmacol 2015;11(7):874–87.
35. Goyal M. Traditional plants used for the treatment of diabetes mellitus in Sursagar constituency, Jodhpur, Rajasthan—an ethnomedicinal survey. J Ethnopharmacol 2015;174:364–8.
36. Nahas R, Moher M. Complementary and alternative medicine for the treatment of type 2 diabetes. Can Fam Physician 2009;55(6):591–6.
37. Kirkham S, Akilen R, Sharma S, et al. The potential of cinnamon to reduce blood glucose levels in patients with type 2 diabetes and insulin resistance. Diabetes Obes Metab 2009;11(12):1100–13.
38. Mooren FC. Magnesium and disturbances in carbohydrate metabolism. Diabetes Obes Metab 2015;17(9):813–23.

39. Pillitteri JL, Shiffman S, Rohay JM, et al. Use of dietary supplements for weight loss in the United States: results of a national survey. Obesity (Silver Spring) 2008;16(4):790–6.

40. Blom WA, Abrahamse SL, Bradford R, et al. Effects of 15-d repeated consumption of Hoodia gordonii purified extract on safety, ad libitum energy intake, and body weight in healthy, overweight women: a randomized controlled trial. Am J Clin Nutr 2011;94(5):1171–81.

41. Geller AI, Shehab N, Weidle NJ, et al. Emergency department visits for adverse events related to dietary supplements. N Engl J Med 2015;373(16):1531–40.

42. Homeopathy. National Center for Complimentary and Integrative Health. Available at: https://nccih.nih.gov/health/homeopathy. Accessed December 1, 2015.

43. The homeopathic pharmacopoeia of the United States. Available at: http://www.hpus.com/what-is-homeopathy.php. Accessed December 1, 2015.

44. USP Verified Dietary Supplements. U.S. Pharmacopoiel convention. Available at: http://www.usp.org/usp-verification-services/usp-verified-dietary-supplements. Accessed December 1, 2015.

Cancer Screening in Older Adults

Ashley H. Snyder, MD[a], Allison Magnuson, DO[b], Amy M. Westcott, MD[c],*

KEYWORDS

- Cancer screening guidelines • Cost • Elderly • High-value care • Life expectancy
- Older adult

KEY POINTS

- Due to the balance between risks and benefits to screening for cancer, an older adult's life expectancy and comorbidities should play a role in deciding when to stop screening for cancer.
- There does not appear to be added value to cancer screening in frail elderly.
- Ongoing conversations between patients/families and clinicians are needed to address cancer screening in the elderly.

INTRODUCTION

When considering the risks and benefits of screening for cancer in the elderly, it is important to remember that screening tests have risks and benefits.[1] Such risks often have more significant consequences in the older adult. As an example, the risks associated with colonoscopy, including bowel perforation, bleeding, diverticulitis, cardiovascular events, and death,[2] all increase with age.[3]

Choosing Wisely is an initiative of the American Board of Internal Medicine (ABIM), which aims to help clinicians and patients choose care that is "supported by evidence, not duplicative of other tests or procedures already received, free from harm and truly necessary." Regarding cancer screening in the elderly, this initiative is in agreement with the American Geriatrics Society's recommendation to not recommend screening for colorectal, prostate, or lung cancer without considering life expectancy and the risks of testing, overdiagnosis, and overtreatment.[4]

Disclosure Statement: The authors have nothing to disclose.
[a] Division of General Internal Medicine, Penn State Milton S. Hershey Medical Center, 500 University Drive, Mail Code H034, Hershey, PA 17033, USA; [b] Division of Hematology/Oncology, Wilmot Cancer Institute, University of Rochester, 601 Elmwood Avenue, Box 704, Rochester, NY 14642, USA; [c] Department of Medicine, Penn State Milton S. Hershey Medical Center, 500 University Drive, Mail Code H106, Hershey, PA 17033, USA
* Corresponding author.
E-mail address: awestcott@hmc.psu.edu

Becker and colleagues[5] describe how as age increases, cancer incidence and cancer-specific mortality rates also increase. They also note that one of the fastest growing segments of the population is the extreme elderly, defined as people 85 years of age and older, with growth in this age category expected to produce at least a fourfold increase in the number of patients with cancer between 2000 and 2050. As the elderly population grows, the impact of cancer screening practices in this population will become increasingly significant, suggesting that special consideration must be given to the concept of high-value care when screening for cancer in older adults.

Because there is a growing population of older adults, it is important to consider the impact of the costs of screening for cancer. Gross and colleagues[6] published a study in 2013 using the linked Surveillance, Epidemiology, and End Results (SEER)–Medicare database from 2006 to 2007 to assess the costs to fee-for-service Medicare for breast cancer screening-related procedures and treatment expenditures. They reported that the cost to Medicare for breast cancer screening in the fee-for-service program exceeds $1 billion dollars annually. For women aged 75 years and older, the cost of breast cancer screening-related procedures exceeded $410 million annually. One year later, O'Donoghue and colleagues[7] reported that in the United States in 2010, with approximately 70% of women screened, the cost of screening mammography was $7.8 billion. Noting controversy regarding the frequency and timing of breast cancer screening, they developed a model to estimate the cost of screening mammography for the year 2010 based on 3 different screening strategies. These strategies included annual screening for women aged 40 to 84 years, biennial screening for women aged 50 to 69 years and biennial screening for women aged 50 to 74 years with personalized discussion for those less than 50 years of age based on risk and for those 75 years and older based on comorbid conditions (US Preventative Services Task Force [USPSTF] guidelines). They reported that the simulated cost of screening 85% of women would be $10.1 billion for women screened annually, $2.6 billion for women screened biennially, and $3.5 billion for women screened according to the USPSTF guidelines. They also found that 2 of the largest drivers of cost were screening frequency and percentage of women screened.

In 2015, Schonberg and colleagues[3] published a study looking at the rates of colorectal cancer screening for years 2008 and 2010 among US adults age 65 years and older based on age and life expectancy, noting that it takes approximately 10 years before 1 death from colorectal cancer is prevented for 1000 individuals screened. They reported that, of the 56% of US adults 65 years of age and older who reported undergoing recent colorectal cancer screening, 28% of those were 75 years of age and older or had a life expectancy of less than 10 years.

Screening in accordance with evidence-based guidelines, while taking into account life expectancy when choosing whom to screen for cancer, is one way to deliver high-value care. This article reviews the 4 common cancers affecting older adults, provides a review of the current screening guidelines for these cancers, and lists the costs of common cancer screening tests. It also explores how clinicians can use life expectancy to better aid in determining who will benefit most from screening. Lastly, it provides tools to help clinicians approach the subject of stopping screening with their older patients.

CANCERS COMMONLY AFFECTING THE ELDERLY

According to data provided by the National Cancer Institute's SEER Program, 52.9% of all new cases of cancer and 69.1% of cancer deaths occurred in people aged

65 years and older between 2008 and 2012.[8] Four major cancers affecting older adults are breast cancer, colorectal cancer, lung cancer, and prostate cancer.[9] **Table 1**, adapted from a table of information provided on the American cancer society (ACS) Web site, shows the estimated number of new cases for each of these types of cancer in adults aged 65 years and older for 2015.[10]

COSTS OF COMMON CANCER SCREENING TESTS

Information regarding the costs of common screening tests can be difficult to find. Web sites such as "healthcarebluebook.com" attempt to make this information more readily available to patients and clinicians by allowing the user to enter their zip code and search for the fair price of common tests and procedures in their area. The site defines the fair price as "the reasonable amount you should pay for a medical service" and notes that it is "calculated from a nationwide database of medical payment data and customized to (the user's) geographic area.[11]"

Table 2 lists the costs for common cancer screening procedures found by entering the zip code of a large, academic, tertiary medical center in central Pennsylvania into the site's search box.[11]

The fair price for common cancer screening tests can vary significantly according to location. This table serves only as a frame of reference for the costs of some common screening tests. Information regarding Medicare reimbursements for common cancer screening tests and procedures can be found at the Centers for Medicare and Medicaid Services Web site (link provided at the end of this article).

USING LIFE EXPECTANCY TO DETERMINE BENEFIT IN CANCER SCREENING

Frailty, comorbidity, and disability are predictive of mortality.[12–15] A comprehensive geriatric assessment can be used to evaluate a patient's overall health status, including comorbidity and frailty, and to develop an estimation of life expectancy. Estimation of life expectancy can be used to determine the potential benefit of therapeutic interventions. For example, if a known intervention has a lag time to benefit of 10 years and a patient has a life expectancy estimation of less than 5 years, the potential risks or adverse effects of that intervention likely outweigh the potential benefits. This concept also can be applied to cancer screening. Cancer screening tools have been evaluated for their lag time to benefit. Lee and colleagues[16] performed a meta-analysis of survival data from the United States, Sweden, United Kingdom, and Denmark to determine pooled estimates of time lags to benefit for breast and colorectal cancer screening across a spectrum of thresholds for

Table 1	
Estimated new cases of the four major cancers in adults 65 years and older	
Cancer Site	**Estimated Number of New Cases in Adults 65 y and Older**
Colon and rectum	80,480
Lung and bronchus	149,700
Breast (women)	99,590
Prostate	126,140

Data from American Cancer Society. Estimated new cases of the four major cancers by sex and age group, 2015. Available at: http://www.cancer.org/acs/groups/content/@editorial/documents/document/acspc-044511.pdf. Accessed November 13, 2015.

Table 2	
Costs for common cancer screening procedures	
Test/Procedure	**Fair Price for 17033 Zip Code**
Colonoscopy	$1795
Occult blood feces, 1–3 tests	$18
Barium enema	$360
Total PSA	$48
Digital bilateral screening mammography	$242
Chest CT (noncontrast)	$309

Data from HealthCareBlueBook. Available at: https://healthcarebluebook.com/. Accessed April 26, 2016.

absolute risk-reduction. Based upon their results, the authors recommended that for patients with a life expectancy of less than 5 years, the risks of colon cancer screening may outweigh the benefits. They also recommended that for patients with a life expectancy less than 3 years, the risks of breast cancer screening may outweigh potential benefits. Lansdorp-Vogelaar and colleagues[17] determined that comorbidity is an important factor of risks and benefits of cancer screening and recommended that comorbidity levels be utilized in decision making for cancer screening as well.

There are several life expectancy estimation tools available for clinicians. Walter and Covinsky[18] used actuarial data to develop life expectancy tables based upon broad health statuses. Authors separated patients into health quartiles, and evaluated the average life expectancy at various ages for the upper 25% health status, lower 25% health status, and middle 50% health status. Several other prognostic indices for life expectancy exist and include measures for unique patient populations and disease groups as well.[19]

REVIEWING CURRENT SCREENING GUIDELINES

This article focuses primarily on the USPSTF and ACS cancer screening guidelines. The current USPSTF guidelines recommend against cervical cancer screening in women older than 65 years of age who have had adequate prior screening and are not at high risk for cervical cancer (D recommendation). Because the authors consider elderly to be persons over the age of 65 years for the purposes of this article, cervical cancer screening guidelines are not discussed in further detail.[20]

Breast Cancer Screening

The USPSTF recommends biennial screening mammography for women aged 50 to 74 years (B recommendation). They report insufficient evidence to assess the additional benefits and harms of screening mammography in women aged 75 years and older (I statement).[21] An update of the USPSTF guidelines for breast cancer screening is currently in progress, but the recommendations in the most recent draft statement are the same as the 2009 recommendations.[22]

For women of average risk, the ACA recommends that women aged 45-54 years should undergo yearly screening mammogram while women aged 40-44 years should be offered the opportunity to begin screening. For women aged 55 years and older, they recommend switching to mammography every 2 years but also recommend that these women be offered the choice for annual mammography. They recommend continued screening as long as the woman is in good health with a life expectancy of 10 years or more.[23]

Colorectal Cancer Screening

The USPSTF recommends screening for colorectal cancer beginning at age 50 years and continuing until age 75 years with fecal occult blood testing, sigmoid-oscopy, or colonoscopy (A recommendation). For adults aged 76 to 85 years, the USPSTF recommends against routine screening for colorectal cancer but suggests that there may be considerations that support screening in individual patients (C recommendation). The USPSTF reports that while the incidence of colorectal cancer increases with age, in individuals who have previously been screened, extending the screening age from 75 years of age to 85 years of age resulted in a small benefit compared with the risks in this age group. For individuals who have never been screened, USPSTF recommends consideration of the individual's overall health status to aid in the decision of whether or not to pursue first time screening, noting that the benefit of screening is typically not seen for 7 years.[2]

Among average-risk individuals, the ACS recommends screening beginning at age 50 with flexible sigmoidoscopy every 5 years, colonoscopy every 10 years, double contrast barium enema every 5 years, or CT colonography every 5 years. ACS recommends stopping screening at a point where curative therapy would not be offered because of life-threatening comorbidity.[24]

Choosing Wisely and the American College of Surgeons recommend avoiding colorectal cancer screening tests on asymptomatic patients with a life expectancy of less than 10 years and no family or personal history of colorectal neoplasia.[4]

Prostate Cancer Screening

The USPSTF reports that 70% of deaths caused by prostate cancer occur after the age of 75 years and, although some cases of prostate cancer are aggressive, most cases have a good prognosis even without treatment and the lifetime risk for dying of prostate cancer is only 2.8%. They cite the potential harms of screening including pain, fever, bleeding, infection, and transient urinary difficulties associated with prostate biopsy, along with potential harms of treatment for prostate cancer, including erectile dysfunction, urinary incontinence, bowel dysfunction, and a small risk for premature death. Citing evidence that the benefits of prostate specific antigen (PSA)-based prostate cancer screening do not outweigh the harms in men of average risk, USPSTF recommends against PSA-based screening, regardless of age, for men of average risk in the US general population (D recommendation).[25]

The current ACS guidelines for prostate cancer screening recommend that patients make an informed decision with their health care provider regarding whether to be screened for prostate cancer. They recommend that this discussion take place at age 50 years for men who are at average risk for the disease and have a life expectancy of at least 10 years, age 45 years for men at high risk for disease (including African Americans and men with a first-degree relative diagnosed with disease at a young age), and at age 40 for men at even higher risk for disease. The ACS guidelines also recommend that men without symptoms of prostate cancer who do not have a 10-year life expectancy should not be offered screening as they are not likely to benefit.[26]

The American Urologic Association (AUA) recommends shared decision making between patient and provider for men aged 55 to 69 years considering PSA-based prostate cancer screening. For men aged 70 years and older or with a life expectancy of

---

Box 1
Steps to communicate discontinuing routine screening

1. Gain understanding of their knowledge base—determine what the patient knows

2. Provide an explanation—provide evidence-based information clearly and avoid medical jargon

3. Acknowledge reaction and provide empathy—example phrase: "It appears that this news may be upsetting to you"

4. Check for understanding and confirm agreement

5. Summarize and discuss reasons why testing would or would not be indicated

---

less than 10 to 15 years, AUA does not recommend routine PSA-based screening. However, there may be potential for benefit from screening in some men older than 70 years who are in excellent health.[27]

Lung Cancer Screening

The USPSTF recommends that adults aged 55 to 80 years with a 30-pack year smoking history who still smoke or who have quit within the past 15 years undergo annual screening for lung cancer with low-dose computed tomography (CT) scan. It is recommended that screening should be discontinued once a person has not smoked for 15 years or the person develops a health problem that substantially limits life expectancy or the ability or willingness to have curative surgery. This was a significant change from the 2004 recommendation, which said that there was insufficient evidence for or against lung cancer screening.[28]

The most current ACS guidelines regarding lung cancer screening are based on the criteria from the National Lung Screening Trial (NLST) and recommend that patients be screened for lung cancer with yearly low-dose CT scan if they are aged 55 to 74 years, are in fairly good health (ability to have surgery or other therapy, no other serious medical problems, not requiring home oxygen), have at least a 30-pack year smoking history and are still smoking or have quit within the last 15 years.[29,30]

Choosing Wisely and the American Geriatrics Society report that much of the evidence for benefit from low-dose CT screening for lung cancer in smokers is from healthier patients under age 65 years. They also report that screening 1000 persons would avoid 4 lung cancer deaths in 6 years but would produce 273 persons with an abnormal result, requiring 36 to get an invasive procedure, with 8 of those suffering complications.[4]

HAVING THE DISCUSSION

Having the discussion with patients about whether to continue screening for cancer based on risks, benefits, and life expectancy can often be challenging. Based on a combination of strategies, including the S-P-I-K-E-S strategy[31] (Buckman 2005), the American Gastroenterological Association's communication module on the Choosing Wisely site[32] (Drossman 2013), and Back and colleagues[33] (Back et al 2009) discussing prognosis, the authors recommend the strategy presented in **Box 1** for initiating the discussion to stop screening with elderly patients.

Presented subsequently is an example of dialogue that can be used between patient and clinician regarding the discussion to stop screening.

Example dialogue

Your patient is an 80-year-old woman who resides in a long-term care community and is dependent for all Activities of Daily Living (ADLs). She has a significant past medical history of depression, atrial fibrillation, and type 2 diabetes mellitus. She presents today for her annual wellness examination.

Patient – "I think I am due to have my annual mammogram done. It has been a couple of years since my last one."

Clinician – "You are right. You had one 3 years ago, and it was normal. So, what do you know about mammograms and breast cancer screening?

Patient – "I know that the mammograms are designed to detect cancers in an early stage before I can feel a lump."

Clinician – "Right again! The only thing I might add is that it may take many years to realize the benefits of periodic mammograms, and patients with multiple medical problems or advanced age may not be around long enough to realize these benefits. Given your age and ongoing medical issue, you are likely one of those folks that will not benefit from continued screening with mammograms. In fact, some guidelines recommend that we stop screening mammograms at age 75."

Patient – "Well, what is the harm of just continuing getting mammograms?"

Clinician – "Great question! If mammograms after age 75 have not been shown to prolong life, then the risks of the biopsies and treatments for abnormal mammograms would outweigh any potential benefits to you. You may want to consider not having any more mammograms. What are your thoughts about this?"

Patient – "I would be OK with stopping. If they discovered cancer, I am not sure I would even want to have any treatments for it anyway."

MAKING AN EVIDENCED-BASED, HIGH-VALUE CANCER SCREENING DECISION: AN EXAMPLE

Mr AT is a 76-year-old patient who is evaluated for his annual examination. He has a history of oxygen-dependent chronic obstructive pulmonary disease (COPD), coronary artery disease, and stage 3 chronic kidney disease. He has never been screened for colon cancer and wonders if this is something he should pursue. On further discussion, you learn that Mr AT has been hospitalized twice in the past 6 months for COPD exacerbation. He currently resides in an assisted living facility and notes difficulty ambulating to the dining room for meals due to dyspnea. He has ADL limitations, and his son assists him with bathing. Per his record, you note he has lost weight over the past 6 months, approximately 12 pounds total. Based upon his significant comorbidity and disability, you determine that he is overall frail and likely has a life expectancy of less than 5 years. You recall the USPSTF guideline recommendation to consider the individual's overall health status when deciding whether to pursue first-time screening, because the benefit of screening is typically not seen for 7 years.[2] Noting his oxygen-dependent COPD, you also recall the ACS recommendation that screening be stopped at a point where curative therapy would not be offered due to life threatening comorbidity.[24] Therefore, you discuss with Mr AT that the benefits of colorectal cancer screening do not outweigh the risks for him and recommend against colorectal cancer screening.

SUMMARY

With over 50% of all new cases of cancer and nearly 70% of all cancer deaths occurring in people aged 65 years and older,[5,8] it is becoming increasingly important to consider the impact of screening for cancer in this population. Value can be defined as the ratio of benefit to cost. In order to maximize the value in screening for cancer in older adults, it is important to screen those who will benefit most.[6,7] By screening in accordance with guidelines and using life expectancy to help choose which patients will benefit most from screening, one can deliver high-value care, the right care delivered at the right time.

HELPFUL LINKS FOR CLINICIANS

Information on PSA: http://www.choosingwisely.org/patient-resources/psa-test-for-prostate-cancer/

Health check-ups: http://www.choosingwisely.org/patient-resources/health-checkups/

Health care blue book: https://healthcarebluebook.com/

Medicare prices for tests: https://www.cms.gov/apps/physician-fee-schedule/

Procedure codes for tests: http://www.hipaaspace.com/Medical_Billing/Coding/Healthcare_Common_Procedure_Coding_System/HCPCS_Codes_Lookup.aspx

USPSTF grade definitions: http://www.uspreventiveservicestaskforce.org/Page/Name/grade-definitions

REFERENCES

1. Soung MC. Screening for cancer: when to stop?: A practical guide and review of the evidence. Med Clin North Am 2015;99(2):249–62.
2. U.S. Preventive Services Task Force. Screening for colorectal cancer: U.S. preventive services task for recommendation statement. Ann Intern Med 2008;149: 627–38.
3. Schonberg MA, Breslau ES, Hamel MB, et al. Colon cancer screening in U.S. adults aged 65 and older according to life expectancy and age. J Am Geriatr Soc 2015;63(4):750–6.
4. American geriatrics society breast colorectal prostate cancer screening in older adults. 2015. Available at: http://www.choosingwisely.org/clinician-lists/american-geriatrics-society-breast-colorectal-prostate-cancer-screening-in-older-adults/. Accessed November 4, 2015.
5. Becker D, Ryemon S, Gross J, et al. Cancer trends among the extreme elderly in the era of cancer screening. J Geriatr Oncol 2014;5(4):408–14.
6. Gross CP, Long JB, Ross JS, et al. The cost of breast cancer screening in the Medicare population. JAMA Intern Med 2013;173(3):220–6.
7. O'Donoghue C, Eklund M, Ozanne EM, et al. Aggregate cost of mammography screening in the United States: comparison of current practice and advocated guidelines. Ann Intern Med 2014;160(3):145–53.
8. SEER stat fact sheets: all cancer sites. 2015. Available at: http://seer.cancer.gov/statfacts/html/all.html. Accessed November 13, 2015.
9. Common cancer types. 2015. Available at: http://www.cancer.gov/types/common-cancers. Accessed November 20, 2015.
10. Estimated new cases of the four major cancers by sex and age group, 2015. 2015. Available at: http://www.cancer.org/acs/groups/content/@editorial/documents/document/acspc-044511.pdf. Accessed November 13, 2015.

11. Healthcare blue book. 2015. Available at: https://healthcarebluebook.com/. Accessed November 7, 2015.
12. Fried LP, Kronmal RA, Newman AB, et al. Risk factors for 5-year mortality in older adults: the Cardiovascular Health Study. JAMA 1998;279(8):585–92.
13. Inouye SK, Studenski S, Tinetti ME, et al. Geriatric syndromes: clinical, research, and policy implications of a core geriatric concept. J Am Geriatr Soc 2007;55(5): 780–91.
14. Fried LP, Tangen CM, Walston J, et al. Frailty in older adults: evidence for a phenotype. J Gerontol A Biol Sci Med Sci 2001;56(3):M146–56.
15. Reuben DB, Rubenstein LV, Hirsch SH, et al. Value of functional status as a predictor of mortality: results of a prospective study. Am J Med 1992;93(6):663–9.
16. Lee SJ, Boscardin WJ, Stijacic-Cenzer I, et al. Time lag to benefit after screening for breast and colorectal cancer: meta-analysis of survival data from the United States, Sweden, United Kingdom, and Denmark. BMJ 2013;346:e8441.
17. Lansdorp-Vogelaar I, Gulati R, Mariotto AB, et al. Personalizing age of cancer screening cessation based on comorbid conditions: model estimates of harms and benefits. Ann Intern Med 2014;161(2):104–12.
18. Walter LC, Covinsky KE. Cancer screening in elderly patients: a framework for individualized decision making. JAMA 2001;285(21):2750–6.
19. Yourman LC, Lee SJ, Schonberg MA, et al. Prognostic indices for older adults: a systematic review. JAMA 2012;307(2):182–92.
20. Final recommendation statement: cervical cancer: screening. 2012. Available at: http://www.uspreventiveservicestaskforce.org/Page/Document/Recommendation StatementFinal/cervical-cancer-screening. Accessed November 20, 2015.
21. US Preventive Services Task Force. Screening for Breast Cancer: U.S. Preventive Services Task Force recommendation statement. Ann Intern Med 2009;151(10):716–26.
22. Breast Cancer Screening Draft Recommendations. 2015. Available at: http://screeningforbreastcancer.org/. Accessed November 6, 2015.
23. American Cancer Society recommendations for early breast cancer detection in women without breast symptoms. 2015. Available at: http://www.cancer.org/cancer/breastcancer/moreinformation/breastcancerearlydetection/breast-cancer-early-detection-acs-recs. Accessed November 6, 2015.
24. Colorectal Cancer Screening and Surveillance Guidelines: Comparison of 2008 ACS/USMSTF/ACR Guidelines with those of the USPSTF. 2014. Available at: http://www.cancer.org/healthy/informationforhealthcareprofessionals/colonmd clinicansinformationsource/colorectalcancerscreeningandsurveillanceguidelines/comparison-of-colorectal-screening-guidelines. Accessed October 28, 2015.
25. Moyer VA. Screening for Prostate Cancer: U.S. Preventive Services Task Force recommendation statement. Ann Intern Med 2012;157(2):120–34.
26. American Cancer Society Recommendations for Prostate Cancer Early Detection. 2015. Available at: http://www.cancer.org/cancer/prostatecancer/moreinformation/prostatecancerearlydetection/prostate-cancer-early-detection-acs-recommendations. Accessed November 6, 2015.
27. Carter HB, Albertsen PC, Barry MJ, et al. Early detection of prostate cancer: AUA Guideline. J Urol 2013;190(2):419–26.
28. Moyer VA. Screening for lung cancer: U.S. Preventive Services Task Force recommendation statement. Ann Intern Med 2014;160(5):330–8.
29. American Cancer Society guidelines for lung cancer screening. 2015. Available at: http://www.cancer.org/cancer/lungcancer-non-smallcell/moreinformation/lung cancerpreventionandearlydetection/lung-cancer-prevention-and-early-detection-guidelines. Accessed November 9, 2015.

30. Smith RA, Manassaram-Baptiste D, Brooks D, et al. Cancer screening in the United States, 2015: a review of current American Cancer Society guidelines and current issues in cancer screening. CA Cancer J Clin 2015;65(1):30–54.
31. Buckman R. Breaking bad news: the S-P-I-K-E-S strategy. Community Oncol 2005;2(2):138–42.
32. Drossman D. The American Gastroenterological Association's Choosing Wisely® Communication Module. 2013. Available at: http://modules.choosingwisely.org/modules/m_04/default_FrameSet.htm. Accessed November 8, 2015.
33. Back A, Arnold R, Tulsky J. Chapter 5: discussing prognosis. Mastering communication with seriously ill patients. New York: Cambridge University Press; 2009. p. 8.

Symptom Control at the End of Life

Margaret Kreher, MD

KEYWORDS

- End of life • Communication • Symptoms • Evidence • Primary palliative care

KEY POINTS

- High-quality end-of-life care begins with good communication. Basic patient-centered assessments and interventions for patients at the end of life are within the purview of primary care physicians.
- The patient's goals are the guide to the application of best practice interventions in providing high value care.

INTRODUCTION

The provision of end-of-life care has become a critically important skill as the population ages. Many people die of a progressive illness that occurs over weeks, months, or years.[1] It is estimated that more than 50% of individuals who die, die with moderate to severe symptoms.[2] The National Consensus Project for Quality Palliative Care and the Institute of Medicine Committee on Approaching Death have identified high-quality practices for end-of-life care.[1,3] High-value end-of-life care demands a holistic approach consistent with the quality practice domains that encompass the physical, psychosocial, and spiritual aspects of care. Despite the introduction of curricula in end-of-life care in medical schools and improvements in access to hospice and palliative care, barriers remain for effective symptom management at the end of life.[1] Access to specialty palliative care is challenged by the supply of physicians certified in the specialty.[4] To meet demand, primary care providers should be educated in the basic principles of symptom management for patients with serious illness.[5] These principles include symptom assessment, alignment of treatment plans with patient's goals, and intervention for suffering in all its domains.[6] This article provides a framework for end-of-life symptom management for providers who are at the front lines of caring. Included in this article are the following:

- Patient-centered end-of-life care
- Communication in serious illness

Disclosure: The author has nothing to disclose.
Department of Medicine, Center of Excellence in Palliative Medicine, Palliative Care, Penn State MS Hershey Medical Center, Mail Code H106, PO Box 850, 500 University Drive, Hershey, PA 17033–0850, USA
E-mail address: mkreher@hmc.psu.edu

Med Clin N Am 100 (2016) 1111–1122
http://dx.doi.org/10.1016/j.mcna.2016.04.020
0025-7125/16/$ – see front matter © 2016 Elsevier Inc. All rights reserved.

- Symptom assessment, management, and burdens of treatment
- Summary and future directions

For the purposes of this article, end of life refers to the final weeks to months before death.

PATIENT-CENTERED END-OF-LIFE CARE

Families' perceptions of their loved-ones' health care providers play an important role in their perceptions of quality of care.[7] Trust of providers, clarity and consistency of information communicated by providers, and ability to engage in decision making with providers is consistently rated highly by patients.[8] Communication has been shown to play a key role in quality-of-life measures by patients with advanced lung cancer receiving concurrent specialist palliative care.[9] It is important to most patients and families to know the prognosis, and to have time to prepare and reconnect and settle unfinished business. The desire for pain and symptom management is linked to the need for time to prepare and reconnect.[10,11] Patient-centeredness has at its core trust, communication, prognostication, preparation, and symptom management.

COMMUNICATION IN SERIOUS ILLNESS

The American College of Physicians High Value Care Task Force conducted a review of evidence regarding communication in serious illness. The task force analyzed the body of mostly qualitative literature regarding communication about serious illness and concluded that patient-centered communication about serious illness and goals of care is a high-value, low-cost intervention.[12] They make the case that high-quality goals-of-care discussions in serious illness are associated with better satisfaction with care, less anxiety, less caregiver distress, care provision that is more congruent with patients' goals, and less nonbeneficial medical interventions at the end of life. Emphasis is also placed on the timing of these conversations. The best time is during a period of stability in the outpatient setting and the worst time is during crisis hospitalization. **Box 1** summarizes key points from the best-practice review.[12]

Box 1
Best practice for communication in serious illness

Patient centered

- Discussion early in the course of serious illness
- Provide information on prognosis, likely course of illness
- Understand patient concerns and goals
- Understand trade-offs patient is willing to make
- Determine family involvement

Health system centered

- Communication skills training for providers
- Triggers for initiating discussions
- Discussion prompts
- Standard documentation that is visible and easily accessed in the electronic health record
- Quality review of discussions with feedback for improvement

SYMPTOM ASSESSMENT, MANAGEMENT, AND BURDENS OF TREATMENT

The 1997 Institute of Medicine report made the case for better end-of-life care.[13] Despite the growth of palliative care and the development of guidelines and quality measures, there is evidence that symptom prevalence measured between 1998 and 2010 has increased. Proxy reports of pain, depression, and delirium in descendants increased over this time period. Whether awareness of symptoms improved or changes in patients or proxies occurred over that time period is not known. However, the need to understand and reverse these trends has been highlighted.[2] Identifying evidence-based best practices in end-of-life care has been challenging because of the vulnerability and heterogeneity of the seriously ill patient populations, cultural and social norms, and variability in practice in end-of-life care.[14]

Despite the challenges of the evidence, there are fundamental symptom-focused interventions in end-of-life care that health care providers should consistently practice. A full history and physical examination, and evaluation of pertinent diagnostic studies, is essential to symptom management at the end of life. Interventions tailored to address the causes of a patient's symptoms should be undertaken when possible. The stage of underlying illness, the patient's prognosis, and the psychosocial and spiritual milieu in which the patient lives should also be considered. Any symptom-driven intervention undertaken should align with the patient's goals of care and reassessments of the efficacy of interventions and adjustments of those interventions should be undertaken.

Common end-of-life symptoms include pain, dyspnea, depression, nausea, vomiting, anxiety, anorexia/cachexia, fatigue, delirium, and spiritual distress. Pain, dyspnea, and fatigue predominate across a variety of advanced diseases.[15] The experience of illness is affected by severity of disease and demographics (eg, financial security), and emotional and social well-being.[16]

The recommendations that follow for symptom control at the end of life can be generalized to the outpatient setting and are directed toward patients whose prognosis is weeks to months. Comfort care for imminently dying hospitalized patients is addressed in a recent review by Blinderman and Billings.[17]

Pain

Pain at the end of life remains a common problem that significantly affects the end-of-life experience.[18] The World Health Organization (WHO) developed guidelines in 1986 for treatment of cancer pain.[19] When the guidelines are used appropriately, it has been estimated that 70% to 100% of patients with cancer can achieve adequate pain control.[20] **Fig. 1** provides a schematic for the usage of nonopioid, opioid, and adjuvant therapies per the WHO guidelines. Pain assessments should be performed at regular intervals. A pain history should include location, onset, duration, quality, severity, and exacerbating or alleviating factors. Most pain syndromes at the end of life are nociceptic, neuropathic, or both. Use of a validated tool and evaluation of patient functional level are also essential components of a pain assessment. Validated assessment tools are available, ranging from the Likert type, to visual analog, to the Wong Baker FACES pain scale (www.WongBakerFACES.org). For patients with advanced dementia, a validated tool such as Pain Assessment in Advanced Dementia (PAINAD) can be used to assess pain severity.[21]

The role of adjuvant (nonopioid) therapy in pain control at the end of life is determined by pain type, prognosis, and specific patient factors. For example, a painful bony metastasis is best treated by single-fraction radiation therapy.[22] Neuropathic pain can be addressed by gabapentin or pregabalin alone or in combination with

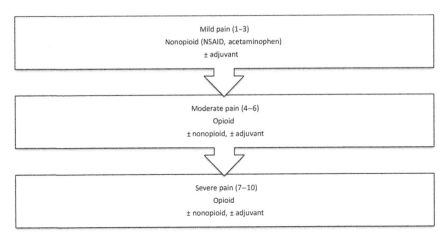

Fig. 1. Hierarchy of pain. NSAID, nonsteroidal antiinflammatory drug.

opioids.[23] **Table 1** outlines various adjuvant interventions.[24] Acetaminophen can be a useful primary analgesic, but it is limited by a maximum dosage of 4 g/d or 2 g/d in patients with liver disease.[25] Nonsteroidal antiinflammatory drugs (NSAIDs) can also be useful in mild to moderate nociceptive pain and as adjuvants with opioid drugs for severe pain caused by bony metastases.[26] NSAIDs may not be tolerated in patients with renal dysfunction or underlying gastritis or peptic ulcer disease. Any patient taking nonsteroidal antiinflammatory agents for greater than 2 weeks should be prescribed proton pump inhibitors to prevent gastritis and ulcers.[27]

The initiation of opioid therapy for moderate to severe pain at the end of life should begin with assessment of unique patient attributes such as end-organ function, age, and pain history. Clinicians should familiarize themselves with a few commonly available opioids and their equianalgesic dosages.[17] **Table 2** provides equianalgesic dosing of commonly used opioids. Usual initial doses are roughly equivalent to 5 to 15 mg of oral morphine equivalents given as needed at 3-hour to 4-hour intervals. Dosage increases are usually recommended to be in 30% to 50% increments. Long-acting opioids should be used for continuous moderate to severe pain in patients requiring multiple daily doses of short-acting opioids.[24] The initial dosage of a long-acting opioid should be approximately 50% to 60% of the calculated total daily short-acting opioid requirement. When a patient is taking long-acting opioids, short-acting opioids should be given as needed at 3-hour to 4-hour intervals for

Table 1 Adjuvant therapies	
Type	**Example**
Procedural	Neural blockade Radiation therapy
Pharmacologic	Nonopioid analgesics, specific drugs to address neuropathic pain
Rehabilitative	Physical/occupational therapy, lymphedema therapy
Psychological	Cognitive-behavior therapy, relaxation therapy
Alternative/ complementary	Massage, acupuncture

Table 2
Common opioid drugs

Opiate	Equianalgesic Dose PO/IV	Comments
Codeine	200 mg/120 mg	Requires conversion via hepatic P450 enzymes to active drug. Genetic variations in its metabolism make its usage less preferable
Morphine	30 mg/10 mg	Liver glucuronidation to M6G and M3G. M6G contributes to opioid effect, M3G is not an opioid and has CNS effects (myoclonus and agitation). Both metabolites require renal clearance and may increase in renal failure
Oxycodone	20 mg/not IV	—
Hydromorphone	7.5 mg/1.5 mg	Liver metabolism, lower concentration of metabolites requiring renal clearance compared with morphine
Fentanyl	NA/100 μg	Liver metabolism to inactive metabolites, useful in renal failure

Abbreviations: CNS, central nervous system; IV, intravenous; NA, not available; PO, by mouth.
  Adapted from Portenoy R, Ahmed E. Principles of opioid use in cancer pain. J Clin Oncol 2014;32:1665.

breakthrough pain. The short-acting dose should be approximately 10% of the total daily dose of the long-acting opioid.[17] Reassessment of pain control is necessary and frequency of reassessment depends on the severity and impact of pain.

The most common side effects of opioid drugs are somnolence and constipation. Somnolence usually improves over days as the patient develops tolerance to this side effect. Constipation is a side effect in which tolerance does not develop and re-quires anticipatory management.[24] Adequate hydration and the prescription of an os-motic agent such as polyethylene glycol or stimulant cathartic such as senna are generally adequate to manage opioid-induced constipation.[28,29] Opioid antagonists such as methyl naltrexone or lubiprostone may be indicated when oral or rectal agents have not been effective in treating constipation.[30] Other common side effects of opioid therapy include nausea, dry mouth, urinary retention, pruritus, and myoclonus.[24] The cost of opioid antagonists can vary, but some of the long-acting preparations are now available in generic form. Generic short-acting and then long-acting opioids can serve as cost-effective first-line and second-line therapies.

Rotating from one opioid to a different opioid may be undertaken when either the route of administration needs to change or the patient is experiencing untoward side effects. Use of an equianalgesic dosing table is needed and a calculation of the equianalgesic dose of the new opioid is performed. Patients may not be tolerant of the side effects of the new opioid and a dose reduction of 25% to 50% of the calcu-lated equianalgesic dosage is required.[24]

Dyspnea

Dyspnea is a subjective experience with both sensory and affective components and assessment should be quantitated by patient rating of severity and/or physical mea-sures.[31] The prevalence of dyspnea at the end of life varies across primary diagnoses and stages of illness. For example, dyspnea at the end of life occurs in 90% of patients with chronic obstructive pulmonary disease (COPD), 70% of patients with lung cancer, and 65% of those with heart failure.[2] Patients with prognoses of greater than weeks stand to benefit from treatment of the underlying cause of the dyspnea, whereas patients who are closer to the end of life may benefit from pure symptom management. **Table 3** outlines modalities for treatment of dyspnea. Supplemental oxygen is a palliative intervention for patients with hypoxemia (Pao_2 <55 mm Hg) and dyspnea. Room air via nasal cannula is as effective as oxygen by nasal cannula in relieving symptoms of dyspnea for patients who are not hypoxemic.[32] Opioids remain the mainstay for all dyspneic patients at the end of life. Typical opioid doses are lower than the doses used for pain.[31]

SPIRITUAL DISTRESS

Attention to the spirituality of patients with advanced cancer has been shown to improve quality of life and is associated with increased use of hospice and with less use of aggressive care at the end of life by patients with high levels of spiritual coping.[33] Nearly 80% of patients with advanced cancers identify 1 or more spiritual concerns. Four spiritual themes dominate:

- Coping practices: how spirituality affects endurance
- Beliefs beyond self: spirituality/religion play an important role in life
- Personal transformation: sense of connection to higher power
- Community relationships: support from spiritual counselors or spiritual community[34]

Physicians, patients, and nurses identify that routine spiritual practices have a positive impact on patients.[35] The National Consensus Panel quality domain of spirituality in end-of-life care has placed addressing spiritual concerns within the purview of physicians and nurses.[3] Simple screening questions could include inquiry into spiritual or religious practices or inquiry into practices that provide the patient with meaning or strength. It is important to identify spiritual distress and initiate interventions through community chaplaincy support or hospital-based chaplaincy support.[36]

Depression

Depression is common symptom affecting up to 60% of patients in the last year of life across a range of illnesses.[2,37] Recognition and treatment of depression are key elements to alleviate this symptom in patients within the last months of life. Psychosocial interventions and pharmacotherapy are mainstay consensus recommendations.[38] The patient's prognosis needs to be considered because of the length of time needed for drugs to take effect. A prognosis of months is needed for patients to benefit from a selective serotonin reuptake inhibitor (SSRI). Psychostimulants should be considered for severe depression when the prognosis is less than 6 months.[36]

Table 3 Targeted interventions for dyspnea	
Underlying Cause	**Treatment**
Effusion	Thoracentesis; pleural catheters for recurrent effusions; pleurodesis
Infection	Antibiotics
COPD	Bronchodilators, oxygen
Heart failure	Diuretics, angiotensin-converting enzyme inhibitors, β-blockers
Tumor obstruction	Bronchial stent

ANXIETY

Anxiety can manifest as a result of several challenges faced by patients at the end of life. Uncertainty of the future and fear of uncontrolled symptoms and death may all contribute to the development of anxiety across the trajectory of illness. Anxiety may be managed through provider support and counseling. However, when it impairs function, both short-term and long-term treatments may be necessary. Cognitive behavior therapy is a recommended modality for treating anxiety. Severe anxiety may be treated by benzodiazepines in the short term and by SSRIs over the longer term (months).[39] Treatment and interventions are related to the degree of impairment related to the severity of the anxiety and the prognosis of the patient.

Fatigue

Fatigue is a prominent symptom reported during the last weeks to months of life in up to 80% of patients.[2] Pharmacologic interventions for cancer-related fatigue have generally been found to have little impact in the symptom of fatigue in patients with advanced cancers. Agents lacking evidence to support usage for fatigue at the end of life include L-carnitine and activating agents (psychostimulants).[40–42] Steroids may be helpful in patients with advanced cancer with fatigue and anorexia. A small study using methylprednisolone versus placebo in patients with advanced cancer showed a statistically significant improvement in fatigue and appetite after 7 days of treatment.[43]

Anorexia/Cachexia

Cachexia is a syndrome that accompanies the end stage of several chronic diseases. It is characterized by a loss of lean body mass, anorexia, increased resting energy expenditures, metabolic alterations, fatigue, and loss of performance status.[44] Several pharmacologic interventions have been studied without demonstrated improvement in cachexia. Appetite stimulants such as progestational agents have short-lived effects and have not shown survival benefits.[36] A phase III trial showed the efficacy of a multidrug diet and nutritional program in improving measures of lean body mass and fatigue in advanced cancers.[44] This trial targeted the different mechanisms involved in the cancer cachexia syndrome and included in its multimodal therapy arm medroxyprogesterone, eicosapentaenoic acid, L-carnitine, and thalidomide along with nutritional supplementation and exercise. The results suggest that the cachexia syndrome is a multifactorial process that likely requires a multifaceted approach to treat. This trial enrolled patients whose prognosis was greater than 4 months and its results may not apply to patients whose prognosis is shorter. It remains to be established whether multidrug treatment in patients with advanced disease is a viable approach to treating anorexia/cachexia.

Anorexia/cachexia syndrome can be associated with family distress, and a lack of knowledge of the role of nutrition and hydration in the last weeks of life is associated with misperceptions of benefit of treatment.[45] Evidence regarding medically assisted hydration in improving quality of life or prolonging life is lacking because of insufficient high-quality studies to establish recommendations.[46] There is evidence to suggest that sedation and myoclonus are improved through hydration and evidence that hydration is associated with fluid retention symptoms. There is no evidence to support the use of artificial nutrition to treat anorexia/cachexia at the end of life. Clinicians need to weigh benefits and burdens of nutrition/hydration in advanced seriously ill patients whose prognoses are short. Decision making regarding the role of hydration and nutrition must be collaborative with the patient and family and consider patient/family goals and beliefs.[17]

Delirium

Delirium is an acute confusional state and may be manifested in an active (agitated) or hypoactive (quiet) manner.[47] It is a common occurrence in patients at the end of life and is associated with patient and family distress, and, when uncontrolled, may prevent death from occurring in the location preferred by the patient.[48] **Fig. 2** outlines the basics of evaluation of and intervention for delirium in patients at the end of life.[36]

Nausea/Vomiting

A mechanistic approach to the evaluation and treatment of nausea and vomiting for patients at the end of life is critical to successful intervention. **Fig. 3** outlines the pathway of nausea and vomiting. The following are the locations of primary receptors in the pathway:

- Gut: chemoreceptors/mechanoreceptors: serotonin type 3 (5HT3)
- Vestibular: histamine type 1 (H1)
- Chemoreceptor trigger zone: dopamine type 2 (D2), 5HT3, neurokinin type 1
- Vomiting center: serotonin type 2, H1

The common causes of nausea in patients at the end of life include constipation, opioids, chemotherapy, and malignant bowel obstruction.[49] Specific agents selected for treatment should target the likely pathway involved. For example, ondansetron is useful for 5HT3-mediated nausea and metoclopramide is useful for D2-mediated nausea. Prokinetic agents, such as metoclopramide, can be helpful in impaired gut motility as well. Haloperidol, a potent D2 antagonist, is often chosen because of its capacity to block chemoreceptor trigger zone–mediated nausea.[49] Steroids should be used for increased intracranial pressure–related nausea and vomiting.[36]

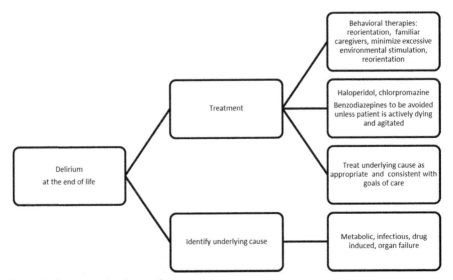

Fig. 2. Delirium: evaluation and treatment.

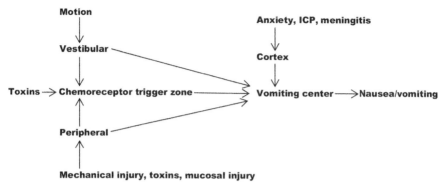

Fig. 3. Nausea/vomiting pathways. ICP, intracranial pressure.

BURDENS OF END-OF-LIFE TREATMENT

Patients at the end of life are at high risk for polypharmacy. In a study of more than 350 hospice patients, potential for therapeutically relevant drug-drug interactions was found in 46% of patients. In addition, the median number of medications prescribed per patient in this study was 10. The most significant adverse effects identified were additive anticholinergic and antidopaminergic toxicities, NSAID-associated toxicity, and QT prolongation.[50] All non–symptom-related medications should be discontinued in patients nearing the end of life. Compounding the challenge of managing symptoms is the lack of robust evidence for several pharmacologic interventions in end-of-life care. The use of antimuscarinics (eg, atropine, glycopyrrolate) for terminal respiratory secretions is based on clinical reports. Systematic review of the evidence has failed to show evidence of efficacy for these drugs.[51] Because of the potential of antimuscarinic side effects, such as delirium, sedation, and xerostomia, routine use of these agents is not recommended in terminal care of patients. However, there may be a rationale for patients with copious oral secretions to attempt a short-term trial of a muscarinic agent.[17] Another example of lack of evidence of efficacy is the use of lorazepam, diphenhydramine, haloperidol (ABH) topical gel for nausea. Testing of drug levels after standard application revealed no therapeutically effective blood levels of any of the combination agents. As part of the American Board of Internal Medicine's Choosing Wisely campaign the American Academy of Hospice and Palliative Medicine Choosing Wisely Task Force recommended that ABH gel not be used until evidence shows effectiveness.[52]

SUMMARY AND FUTURE DIRECTION

Comfort in the last weeks to months of life encompasses the holistic assessment of the patient's suffering and the judicious use of treatment modalities to alleviate suffering and improve quality of life. This article is a broad overview of the holistic approach. The goal is to provide primary providers with a framework for caring. The framework allows patients the opportunity for improved access to basic end-of-life care in the setting of limited numbers of specialty providers. This approach may improve access to services from specialty palliative care teams for patients with complex psychosocial, spiritual, and physical suffering. High-value care depends on high-quality evidence. The challenge of studying the complex questions that exist in the care of patients at the end of life requires the use of valid diverse methodologies to better serve the seriously ill patients and their families for the future delivery of higher-quality and more valuable care.[53]

REFERENCES

1. Dying in America: improving quality and honoring individual preferences near the end of life IOM (Institute of Medicine). 2015.
2. Singer AE, Meeker D, Teno JM, et al. Symptom trends in the last year of life from 1998 to 2010: a cohort study. Ann Intern Med 2015;162(3):175–83.
3. Clinical practice guidelines for quality palliative care. In: Dahlin C, editor. 3rd edition. Pittsburgh: National Consensus Project for Quality Palliative Care; 2013. p. 74.
4. Lupu D, American Academy of Hospice and Palliative Medicine Workforce Task Force. Estimate of current hospice and palliative medicine physician workforce shortage. J Pain Symptom Manage 2010;40(6):899–911.
5. Quill TE, Abernethy AP. Generalist plus specialist palliative care–creating a more sustainable model. N Engl J Med 2013;368(13):1173–5.
6. Ghosh A, Dzeng E, Cheng MJ. Interaction of palliative care and primary care. Clin Geriatr Med 2015;31(2):207–18.
7. Shinjo T, Morita T, Hirai K, et al. Care for imminently dying cancer patients: family members' experiences and recommendations. J Clin Oncol 2010;28(1):142–8.
8. Heyland D, Dodek P, Rocker G, et al. What matters most in end-of-life care: perceptions of seriously ill patients and their family members. CMAJ 2006;174(5):9.
9. Jacobsen J, Jackson V, Dahlin C, et al. Components of early palliative care consultation in patients with metastatic non-small cell lung cancer. J Palliat Med 2011;14(4):459–64.
10. Steinhauser K, Clipp E, McNeilly M, et al. Search of a good death: observations of patients, families and providers. Ann Intern Med 2000;132:825–32.
11. Steinhauser K, Christakis N, Clipp E, et al. Preparing for the end-of-life: preferences of patients, families, physicians and other care providers. J Pain Symptom Manage 2001;22:727–37.
12. Bernacki R, Block S. Communication about serious illness care goals a review and synthesis of best practices. JAMA Intern Med 2014;174(12):1994–2003.
13. Field MJ, Cassel CK, editors. Approaching death: improving care at the end of life. Washington, DC: Institute of Medicine; 1997.
14. Aoun S, Nekolaichuk C. Improving the evidence base in palliative care to inform practice and policy: thinking outside the box. J Pain Symptom Manage 2014; 48(6):1222–34.
15. Solano JP, Gomes B, Higginson IJ. A comparison of symptom prevalence in far advanced cancer, AIDS, heart disease, chronic obstructive pulmonary disease and renal disease. J Pain Symptom Manage 2006;31(1):58–69.
16. Steinhauser KE, Arnold RM, Olsen MK, et al. Comparing three life-limiting diseases: does diagnosis matter or is sick, sick? J Pain Symptom Manage 2011;42(3):331–41.
17. Blinderman C, Billings J. Comfort care for patients dying in the hospital. N Engl J Med 2015;373(26):2549–61.
18. Smith AK, Cenzer IS, Knight SJ, et al. The epidemiology of pain during the last 2 years of life. Ann Intern Med 2010;153(9):563–9.
19. World Health Organization. Traitement de la douleur cancéreuse. Geneva (Switzerland): World Health Organization; 1987.
20. Meuser T, Pietruck C, Radbruch L, et al. Symptoms during cancer pain treatment following WHO-guidelines: a longitudinal follow-up study of symptom prevalence, severity and etiology. Pain 2001;93:247–57.

21. Warden V, Hurley AC, Volicer L. Development and psychometric evaluation of the Pain Assessment in Advanced Dementia (PAINAD) scale. J Am Med Dir Assoc 2003;4(1):9–15.

22. Lutz S, Berk L, Chang E, et al. Palliative radiotherapy for bone metastases: an ASTRO evidence-based guideline. Int J Radiat Oncol Biol Phys 2011;79(4):965–76.

23. Gilron I, Bailey JM, Tu D, et al. Morphine, gabapentin, or their combination for neuropathic pain. N Engl J Med 2005;352(13):1324–34.

24. Portenoy R, Ahmed E. Principles of opioid use in cancer pain. J Clin Oncol 2014;32:1662–70.

25. Bosilkovska M, Walder B, Besson M, et al. Analgesics in patients with hepatic impairment: pharmacology and clinical implications. Drugs 2012;72(12):1645–69.

26. Groninger H, Vijayam J. Pharmacologic management of pain at the end of life. Am Fam Physician 2014;90(1):26–32.

27. American Geriatrics Society Panel on the Pharmacological Management of Persistent Pain in Older Persons. Pharmacological management of persistent pain in older persons. J Am Geriatr Soc 2009;57:1331–46.

28. Lee-Robichaud H, Thomas K, Morgan J, et al. Lactulose versus polyethylene glycol for chronic constipation. Cochrane Database Syst Rev 2010;(7):CD007570.

29. Ford AC, Brenner DM, Schoenfeld PS. Efficacy of pharmacological therapies for the treatment of opioid-induced constipation: systematic review and meta-analysis. Am J Gastroenterol 2013;108(10):1566–74 [quiz: 1575].

30. Becker G, Galandi D, Blum HE. Peripherally acting opioid antagonists in the treatment of opiate-related constipation: a systematic review. J Pain Symptom Manage 2007;34(5):547–65.

31. Mahler DA, Selecky PA, Harrod CG, et al. American College of Chest Physicians consensus statement on the management of dyspnea in patients with advanced lung or heart disease. Chest 2010;137(3):674–91.

32. Abernathy A, McDonald C, Frith P, et al. Effect of palliative oxygen versus room air in relief of breathlessness in patients with refractory dyspnoea: a double-blind, randomised controlled trial. Lancet 2010;376(9743):784–93.

33. Balboni TA, Paulk ME, Balboni MJ, et al. Provision of spiritual care to patients with advanced cancer: associations with medical care and quality of life near death. J Clin Oncol 2010;28(3):445–52.

34. Alcorn SR, Balboni MJ, Prigerson HG, et al. "If God wanted me yesterday, I wouldn't be here today": religious and spiritual themes in patients' experiences of advanced cancer. J Palliat Med 2010;13(5):581–8.

35. Phelps AC, Lauderdale KE, Alcorn S, et al. Addressing spirituality within the care of patients at the end of life: perspectives of patients with advanced cancer, oncologists, and oncology nurses. J Clin Oncol 2012;30(20):2538–44.

36. Kelley AS, Morrison RS. Palliative care for the seriously Ill. N Engl J Med 2015;373(8):747–55.

37. Walker J, Holm Hansen C, Martin P, et al. Prevalence of depression in adults with cancer: a systematic review. Ann Oncol 2013;24(4):895–900.

38. Qaseem A, Snow V, Shekelle P, et al. Evidence-based interventions to improve the palliative care of pain, dyspnea and depression at the end of life: a clinical practice guideline form the American College of Physicians. Ann Intern Med 2008;148:141–6.

39. Traeger L, Greer JA, Fernandez-Robles C, et al. Evidence-based treatment of anxiety in patients with cancer. J Clin Oncol 2012;30(11):1197–205.

40. Cruciani RA, Zhang JJ, Manola J, et al. L-carnitine supplementation for the management of fatigue in patients with cancer: an eastern cooperative oncology group phase III, randomized, double-blind, placebo-controlled trial. J Clin Oncol 2012;30(31):3864–9.
41. Spathis A, Fife K, Blackhall F, et al. Modafinil for the treatment of fatigue in lung cancer: results of a placebo-controlled, double-blind, randomized trial. J Clin Oncol 2014;32(18):1882–8.
42. Mitchell GK, Hardy JR, Nikles CJ, et al. The effect of methylphenidate on fatigue in advanced cancer: an aggregated N-of-1 trial. J Pain Symptom Manage 2015; 50(3):289–96.
43. Paulsen O, Klepstad P, Rosland J, et al. Efficacy of methylprednisolone on pain, fatigue and appetite loss in patients with advanced cancer using opioids: a randomized, placebo-controlled, double-blind trial. J Clin Oncol 2014;32(29): 3221–8.
44. Mantovani G, Maccio A, Madeddu C, et al. Randomised phase III clinical trial of five different arms of treatment in 332 patients with cancer cachexia. Oncologist 2010;15(2):200–11.
45. Del Rio MI, Shand B, Bonati P, et al. Hydration and nutrition at the end of life: a systematic review of emotional impact, perceptions, and decision-making among patients, family, and health care staff. Psychooncology 2012;21(9):913–21.
46. Good P, Richard R, Syrmis W, et al. Medically assisted hydration for adult palliative care patients. Cochrane Database Syst Rev 2014;(4):CD006273.
47. Spiller J, Keen JC. Hypoactive delirium: assessing the extent of the problem for inpatient specialist palliative care. Palliat Med 2006;20(1):17–23.
48. Breitbart W, Alici Y. Agitation and delirium at the end of life: "We couldn't manage him". JAMA 2008;300(24):2898–910.
49. Wood G, Shega J, Lynch B, et al. Management of intractable nausea and vomiting at the end of life "I was feeling nauseous all of the time...nothing was working". JAMA 2007;298(10):1196–207.
50. Frechen S, Zoeller A, Ruberg K, et al. Drug interactions in dying patients: a retrospective analysis of hospice inpatients in Germany. Drug Saf 2012;35(9): 745–58.
51. Wee B, Hillier R. Interventions for noisy breathing in patients near to death. Cochrane Database Syst Rev 2008;(1):CD005177.
52. Fischberg D, Bull J, Casarett D, et al. Five things physicians and patients should question in hospice and palliative medicine. J Pain Symptom Manage 2013; 45(3):595–605.
53. Visser C, Hadley G, Wee B. Reality of evidence-based practice in palliative care. Cancer Biol Med 2015;12(3):193–200.

Treating Dyspnea
Is Oxygen Therapy the Best Option for All Patients?

 CrossMark

Jennifer Baldwin, MD*, Jaclyn Cox, DO

KEYWORDS

- Dyspnea • Breathlessness • Hypoxia • Supplemental oxygen • End-of-life care
- Palliative care

KEY POINTS

- There is a high prevalence of dyspnea at or near the end of life that is associated with significant health and economic burden.
- The mechanism of dyspnea is complex and varies among disease entities and patient experience, making assessment and management challenging.
- Given the anxiety, social isolation, and poor quality of life associated with dyspnea, management is essential and should be tailored to individual patients and their disease.
- Oxygen therapy has been shown to improve survival in patients with COPD with severe hypoxemia, but further research is needed to understand the role of oxygen in moderate and exertional hypoxemia.
- No clear role for supplemental oxygen in the treatment of dyspnea in patients with no hypoxemia has been established, and providers should consider the negative effects of oxygen supplementation. In some instances, symptom control with medications (especially opioids), exercise, behavioral therapy, treatment of associated anxiety, and even the use of fans may be more effective and less costly than oxygen therapy.

INTRODUCTION

In 1999, the American Thoracic Society defined dyspnea as "a subjective experience of breathing discomfort that consists of qualitatively distinct sensations varying in intensity. The experience derives from interactions among multiple physiologic, psychological, social, and environmental factors."[1] This complex sensation of breathlessness is common among many disease entities and is not limited to pulmonary, cardiac, or neuromuscular diseases.

The authors have no commercial or financial conflicts of interest to report. They have no funding sources for this project.
University of Connecticut, 263 Farmington Avenue, Farmington, CT 06032, USA
* Corresponding author.
E-mail address: jbaldwin@uchc.edu

Med Clin N Am 100 (2016) 1123–1130
http://dx.doi.org/10.1016/j.mcna.2016.04.018
0025-7125/16/$ – see front matter © 2016 Elsevier Inc. All rights reserved.

medical.theclinics.com

Many patients in the advanced stages of disease suffer from dyspnea; its prevalence and intensity increase as death approaches.[2] Dyspnea affects many dimensions of a patient's life, reduces activity levels and functional capacity, and causes distress and discomfort. The breathlessness that characterizes many advanced diseases often remains untreatable, adding significant distress to patients and caregivers. It is often associated with depression, anxiety, fear, and social isolation.[3]

More than half a million patients in the United States die annually from diseases that cause dyspnea, and some patients suffer for many years with this symptom.[4] A total of 94% of patients with chronic obstructive pulmonary disease (COPD), 50% of patients with heart failure, and 90% of patients with lung cancer experience dyspnea.[5] Advancing treatments of chronic diseases may often delay, but do not prevent, the onset of dyspnea. As patients live longer, the prevalence and economic burden increases.

It is difficult to determine the exact costs associated with dyspnea. However, a 2011 study found that the average annual all-cause medical costs per patient with COPD and cardiovascular disease was $22,755.[6] Per data from 2010, use of supplemental long-term oxygen therapy (LTOT) by patients with COPD is common, with more than 1 million Medicare recipients using oxygen annually at a cost of more than $2 billion.[7] Despite medical advances in treating chronic diseases and the amount of money spent on patients with these diseases, the ability to treat the accompanied breathlessness has been limited.

PATHOPHYSIOLOGY OF DYSPNEA

Dyspnea is a complex individual experience, and the mechanism is poorly understood, especially when compared with the sensation of pain.[8] Both pain and dyspnea are clearly associated with negative emotions,[9] which can then worsen symptoms, creating a vicious cycle. This perception of dyspnea can vary considerably among patients and is often not explained by disease severity. Previous experiences with dyspnea and a patient's expectations can worsen symptoms.[10]

Mechanism of Dyspnea

There are many causes of the perception of dyspnea in patients. One of the first relates to true airflow obstruction and an increase in mechanical impedance.[11] This resistance to airflow can be related to obstruction and hyperinflation as seen in patients which COPD, effusions, endobronchial lesions, or parenchymal infiltrates. Respiratory muscles that allow chest wall expansion and lung inflation may also not be able to match the input they receive from their own mechanical receptors, vagal receptors in the airways and lungs, or extrathoracic receptors on the face or in the central nervous system.

Other causes of dyspnea include increased ventilatory demand causing increased minute ventilation, such as during physical activity. In patients with COPD, a disruption of physiologic balance, such as increased CO_2 production or lactic acidosis, increases their drive to breathe. Respiratory muscle function itself may also decrease in patients with lung hyperinflation and neuromuscular disease. Anxiety can also provoke dyspnea through increased central perception, perhaps explaining why past experience and memory can trigger symptoms for patients.[11]

Symptoms of Dyspnea

Patients describe dyspnea in various ways, including a sensation of being suffocated or of impending death. Patients may describe an inability to get in enough air or chest tightness. They may experience shallow breathing or decreased respiratory effort related to muscle weakness and fatigue. It is often difficult for patients to distinguish dyspnea from pain, fatigue, loss of energy, or weakness. They may experience pain with breathing, be tired by the effort of breathing, or have anxiety that they interpret as dyspnea.[12]

Dyspnea is sensed through central and peripheral chemoreceptors in response to increased $Paco_2$, decreased Pao_2, or decreased pH, although these are highly variable among patients. Some patients describe dyspnea even with a normal Pao_2, whereas others may not be dyspneic even with a low Pao_2.[13]

MANAGEMENT GOALS AND TREATMENT OPTIONS: REDUCING DYSPNEA AND IMPROVING QUALITY OF LIFE

The goal of treatment is to decrease the perception of dyspnea to improve quality of life. There is some evidence that this can be accomplished by improving exercise tolerance and endurance. Other strategies include use of various medications (especially opioids), smoking cessation, supplemental oxygen therapy, stimulating airflow, and/or suctioning to remove secretions.[11] Certain treatment options are more appropriate for some patients than for others, and understanding the pathophysiology of an individual patient's dyspnea helps identify the best treatment. When dyspnea is related to a mechanism that decreases mechanical impedance (eg, in COPD or lung cancer), there are many different treatment options other than supplemental oxygen. In COPD, inhaled β-agonists and/or anticholinergics and inhaled and systemic steroids can help alleviate obstruction and symptoms. β-Agonists, both long- and short-acting, can induce airway muscle relaxation in the small airways. Inhaled anticholinergics work in a similar way on the larger airways and bronchi. Steroids are used as anti-inflammatories for the airways and are given by inhalation or systemically. Systemic steroids, however, can worsen muscle weakness and cause immunosuppression. Anticholinergics can also be used systemically in the form of patches or liquid drops; however, these are often used only during end-of-life care to decrease secretions. Suction catheters may help physically remove secretions from the airway providing relief. In lung cancer steps may be taken to alleviate symptoms related to collapsed airways, such as bronchial stents. Malignant effusions are managed through frequent drainage by thoracentesis, permanent drain placement, or pleurodesis.[11]

When dyspnea is related to a decrease in ventilatory demand, symptoms can be improved by engaging in exercises to decrease muscle fatigue and weakness thereby decreasing minute ventilation. These exercises and activities are an important part of pulmonary rehabilitation programs for patients with COPD.

The use of opioids in alleviating dyspnea is controversial, mainly because of safety concerns in the nonpalliative patient due to respiratory depression. Opioids work in alleviating the symptom of dyspnea by reducing the ventilator response to the factors that drive dyspnea, such as hypoxia or increased CO_2. They have also been shown to reduce oxygen consumption leading to the decrease in "air hunger."[13] Opioids and benzodiazapines, which act as anxiolytics, may also provide relief by decreasing the central perception of symptoms. Increased airflow may also work to decrease this perception and is discussed in further management options of patient's without hypoxemia.

Pulmonary rehabilitation has been shown to improve dyspnea, fatigue, and functional exercise capacity in patients with COPD.[12] Exercise, coupled with cognitive and behavioral programs, seems to lower dyspnea-related anxiety more than dyspnea itself. By improving anxiety, the perception of dyspnea improves without actually altering the underlying disease process. This is also beneficial because as anxiety levels and perception of dyspnea increase the quality of life suffers. In addition, costs rise as patients take more medications, schedule more office visits with their health care providers, and visit the emergency department more often. Therefore, exercise can desensitize a patient to breathlessness and lessen their fears.

Anecdotally, patients have reported using a fan or standing in front of an open window alleviates their breathlessness.[14] More recently, there is a growing body of evidence to suggest that fans provide symptomatic relief by providing facial airflow. The cooling and/or airflow stimulation of the skin and mucosae innervated by the second and third branches of the trigeminal nerve is thought to be the mechanism of action.[15] Fans are an inexpensive, safe, and portable way to manage dyspnea. Portability and safety are paramount to providing comprehensive symptom relief in palliative care.

Dyspnea Secondary to Hypoxemia

In patients with COPD experiencing severe hypoxemia (Pao_2 <55 mm Hg or Pao_2 <59 mm Hg with signs of right-sided heart strain or polycythemia), LTOT has been shown to improve survival. This was demonstrated in patients with COPD in two randomized controlled trials: the Nocturnal Oxygen Therapy Trial in 1980 and the Medical Research Council study in 1981. Current recommendations for prescribing LTOT are based on the results of these two studies.[16,17]

In the Medical Research Council study, patients with COPD and severe airflow limitation (forced expiratory volume in 1 second, 0.58–0.76 L), severe hypoxemia (Pao_2, 49–52 mm Hg), hypercapnia ($Paco_2$, 53–60 mm Hg), and mild pulmonary hypertension were assigned to at least 2 L/min of oxygen to achieve a Pao_2 greater than 60 mm Hg for 15 hours per day including nocturnal oxygen compared with no LTOT. The trial demonstrated the primary outcome of improved survival with LTOT. There were no differences in pulmonary hemodynamics among secondary outcomes. The 15 hour per day time period was based on reduction of pulmonary arterial pressure.[16]

In the Nocturnal Oxygen Therapy Trial, continuous use of LTOT was compared with nocturnal oxygen therapy in patients with COPD and severe hypoxemia (Pao_2 <56 mm Hg) or moderate hypoxemia (Pao_2 <60 mm Hg) and edema, polycythemia (hematocrit >54%), or right atrial enlargement seen on electrocardiogram (p pulmonale). The relative risk of death for nocturnal oxygen alone was about twice that for continuous LTOT (relative risk, 1.94; 95% confidence interval, 1.17–3.24). In the LTOT group, mean oxygen use was 17.7 hours per day compared with 12 hours per day in the nocturnal oxygen group. Continuous use of LTOT was associated with reduced hematocrit and pulmonary vascular resistance compared with the nocturnal oxygen therapy group.[17]

The results of these two trials demonstrate that some oxygen is better than none in terms of survival in these patients and that continuous oxygen therapy is superior to nocturnal therapy in patients with COPD with hypoxemia at rest. These results have guided the Centers for Medicare and Medicaid Services regarding reimbursement for oxygen therapy. It is still unclear, however, if LTOT improves survival in more moderate hypoxemia (Pao_2, 56–65) and during sleep or exercise. Two separate studies failed to demonstrate that supplemental oxygen improves survival in patients with COPD with moderate hypoxemia, although only small numbers of patients were enrolled.[18]

Oxygen therapy requirements can vary with activity level, and higher amounts of supplemental oxygen may be required during activity. Patients with COPD may also have decreased sensitivity to the normal neurochemical control of breathing during sleep, which can result in nocturnal oxygen desaturation. Subsequently, many patients meet requirements for oxygen therapy at night. Some guidelines recommend increasing the oxygen flow rates during periods of extended exercise and during sleep. Patients often describe difficulty falling asleep, staying asleep, morning tiredness, early awakenings, and excessive daytime sleepiness, but the role of nocturnal oxygen therapy for improving sleep quality in patients with COPD is unknown.[18]

It has been shown that patients with COPD and normal oxygen levels at rest, but low exertional oxygen levels, seem to have a poor prognosis. However, the National Emphysema Treatment Trial failed to demonstrate a benefit among patients who received either continuous, intermittent, or no oxygen therapy.[19] The effect of continuous oxygen therapy in this group of patients with COPD has not been assessed in a prospective trial in a large population.[18]

Short duration, intermittent supplemental oxygen therapy has been used to relieve breathlessness with activity, although there is no uniform definition of the amount or duration of oxygen therapy required. Some studies have shown increased walking distances with supplemental oxygen by increasing endurance time and reducing tachypnea. Published reports have used oxygen to relieve breathlessness, before, during, or after exercise, as needed. A meta-analysis of oxygen therapy found that oxygen augmented the benefits of activity, but noted the limited number of patients and varied study designs.[20]

Dyspnea in the Patient with no Hypoxemia

Despite lack of evidence, it is often considered standard of care for providers to prescribe oxygen for patients who report dyspnea with advanced end-of-life illnesses regardless of Pao_2 levels. In one survey, 70% of providers stated they would prescribe supplemental oxygen for refractory dyspnea and 35% of providers said they would prescribe it on patient or caregiver request despite a lack of hypoxemia.[21] Providers and caregivers often think supplemental oxygen is beneficial whatever the underlying cause and that palliative oxygen is crucial for alleviating suffering. "Compassionate use" oxygen prescribing accounted for 24% of Medicare and Medicaid's budget for LTOT.[21]

A systematic review and meta-analysis published in 2012 found no advantage for supplemental oxygen for alleviating dyspnea in patients with cancer but did find a beneficial effect of opioid treatment. Most trials in this analysis included patients with lung cancer and lung metastases.[22]

A landmark, multicenter, double-blinded, randomized controlled trial demonstrated supplemental oxygen provides no additional benefit for relief of refractory dyspnea in patients with a Pao_2 greater than or equal to 55 mm Hg compared with room air delivered via nasal cannula. In this study, the intensity in which the patient experienced dyspnea improved with oxygen or room air delivered via nasal cannula. Possible reasons for this outcome include symptom relief caused by increased airflow across the nasal passages and the presence of the intervention leading to an improvement in the patients' level of anxiety.[23]

Johnson and coworkers[24] present the current understanding of the use of oxygen compared with "medical air" (ie, compressed room air) for treating refractory breathlessness in advanced disease. They show that of 13 systematic reviews of rigorously designed studies in a variety of patients with cancer, chronic heart failure, kyphoscoliosis, and COPD, 11 failed to demonstrate an incremental benefit of oxygen therapy for treating breathlessness.

Negative Effects of Oxygen Therapy

In addition to the lack of efficacy seen in patients with no hypoxia with LTOT, one also has to consider the negative effects of the therapy. For one, it is burdensome to patients. In one study, only 15% of patients surveyed believed that oxygen therapy was "nonburdensome."[24] In addition, oxygen therapy can be dangerous for patients who rely on their hypoxic drive to ventilate. The literature has also documented significant trauma related to flammability, not only for patients, but also for caregivers who smoke within the home. In addition, patients often report dry nasal passages, and epistaxis can become a significant problem. Oxygen therapy requires installation and monitoring of the concentrator and frequent delivery of new canisters. Patients' homes are often altered to accommodate equipment and electrical usage increases, both of which cause added expense.[24]

Psychological dependence on oxygen therapy can also develop, so if a patient's oxygen malfunctions or the oxygen supply runs out, it may result in an unnecessary health care visit.[24] Oxygen has also been shown to decrease a patient's ability to participate in activities of daily living. Less participation in activities of daily living can worsen quality of life, functional capacity, and exercise tolerance, which in turn can worsen dyspnea. Oxygen therapy can make it more difficult for patients to leave their homes, leading to social isolation. There may be a social stigma associated with oxygen therapy for some patients, which can also worsen isolation.

EVALUATION

When evaluating dyspnea, it is important to consider symptom severity, which may be characterized according to functional status, quality of life, and the underlying disease entity. The question of when to transition from restorative treatment to palliative care is often difficult and varies among patients. It should be considered at least by the time a patient is dyspneic at rest, and all reversible causes of dyspnea have been treated. Clinicians should spend time with their patients making plans for managing their breathlessness including acute hospitalization, mechanical ventilation, or palliative measures. Patients benefit from palliative care even when they are still considering hospitalization and mechanical ventilation. Restorative and palliative management options are not distinct entities and should be used and discussed simultaneously.[11]

Given the subjectivity when measuring a patient's dyspnea in the clinical setting, several tools have been developed to standardize measurement. Most tools for evaluating dyspnea rely on the patient's ability to self-report. Patients closer to death may not be able to report symptoms because of varying levels of consciousness or declining cognition, leading to underrecognition or undertreatment of their symptoms.[25]

The Respiratory Distress Observation Scale is an example of a validated tool to help capture symptoms in patients who are unable to self-report. This scale uses eight observer-rated parameters: (1) heart rate, (2) respiratory rate, (3) accessory muscle use, (4) paradoxic breathing pattern, (5) restlessness, (6) grunting at end-expiration, (7) nasal flaring, and (8) a fearful facial display.[26] During the dying process, when a patient is no longer able to communicate, supplemental oxygen is often used even though there is a lack of evidence for a clear benefit. This can prolong the dying process, thereby increasing distress on the patient and their caregivers, and increasing cost.[27]

FUTURE CONSIDERATIONS/SUMMARY

Oxygen therapy in patients with dyspnea and significant hypoxia has been shown to be an effective intervention. In patients with dyspnea but normal oxygen levels, there is little evidence to suggest a benefit to oxygen therapy. Despite this, many patients receive oxygen (and its associated costs and problems), especially at the end of life. There are numerous effective and high-value approaches to treating dyspnea in the patient with no hypoxemia. Such approaches include medications (eg, opioids and benzodiazepines), fans, compressed air, and pulmonary rehabilitation. Specific guidelines for prescribing supplemental oxygen for the treatment of dyspnea are needed to reduce unnecessary use. Current guidelines are inconsistent, and most allow for a therapeutic trial of palliative oxygen even in patients who do not qualify for LTOT. For example, the National Institute of Health and Clinical Excellence allows for the use of palliative supplemental oxygen to treat breathlessness in patients with COPD. Other published guidelines for treating heart failure acknowledge that there is a lack of evidence to suggest benefit for palliative oxygen, but state that palliative oxygen may be beneficial under certain circumstances. Still other treatment guidelines do not even mention the use of supplemental oxygen.[18]

Johnson and coworkers[24] identify specific areas requiring further research. These include determining.

- How oxygen therapy alleviates breathlessness
- Subgroups of patients who most benefit from oxygen therapy
- The role of palliative oxygen therapy
- Assessing the optimal pattern of use (ie, long-term, nocturnal, and/or short burst oxygen therapy)
- The health and economic cost of palliative oxygen therapy
- Factors that prompt the use of oxygen therapy
- If under certain circumstances oxygen therapy may be deleterious to the patient

It is the goal of health care providers to alleviate suffering for patients and their families. Additional research is clearly needed, but in the meantime providers need to treat patients based on the available evidence and gain a better understanding of the benefit of different therapies for individual patients.

REFERENCES

1. Dyspnea. Mechanisms, assessment, and management: a consensus statement. American Thoracic Society. Am J Respir Crit Care Med 1999;159:321–40.
2. Bausewein C, Booth S, Gysels M, et al. Individual breathlessness trajectories do not match summary trajectories in advanced cancer and chronic obstructive pulmonary disease: results from a longitudinal study. Palliat Med 2010;24:777–86.
3. Bausewein C, Farquhar M, Booth S, et al. Measurement of breathlessness in advanced disease: a systematic review. Respir Med 2007;101:399–410.
4. Solano JP, Gomes B, Higginson IJ. A comparison of symptom prevalence in far advanced cancer, AIDS, heart disease, chronic obstructive pulmonary disease and renal disease. J Pain Symptom Manage 2006;31:58–69.
5. Edmonds P, Karslen S, Khan S, et al. A comparison for the palliative care needs of patients dying from chronic respiratory diseases and lung cancer. Palliat Med 2001;15:287–329.
6. Dalal A, Shah M, Lunacsek O, et al. Clinical and economic burden of patients diagnosed with COPD with comorbid cardiovascular disease. Respir Med 2011;105(10):1516–22.
7. Croxton TL, Bailey WC. Long-term oxygen treatment in chronic obstructive pulmonary disease: recommendations for future research: an NHLBI workshop report. Am J Respir Crit Care Med 2006;1744:373–8.

8. Hayen A, Herigstad M, Pattinson K. Understanding dyspnea as a complex individual experience. Maturitas 2013;76:45–50.
9. Von Leupolt A, Sommer T, Kegat S, et al. Dyspnea and pain share emotion-related brain network. Neuroimage 2009;48:200–6.
10. Mahler DA, Harver A, Lentine T, et al. Descriptors of breathlessness in cardiopulmonary cardiorespiratory and NOT cardiopulmonary diseases. Am J Respir Crit Care Med 1996;154(5):1357–63.
11. Luce JM, Luce JA. Management of dyspnea in patients with far advanced lung disease. JAMA 2001;285(10):1331–7.
12. Herigstad M, Hayen A, Wiech K, et al. Dyspnea and the brain. Respir Med 2011; 105:809–17.
13. Uronis HE, Currow DC, Abernethy AP. Palliative management of refractory dyspnea in COPD. Int J Chron Obstruct Pulmon Dis 2006;1(3):289–304.
14. Galbraith S, Fagan P, Perkins P, et al. Does the use of a handheld fan improve chronic dyspnea? A randomized, controlled, crossover trial. J Pain Symptom Manage 2010;39:831–8.
15. Booth S, Gailbraith S, Ryan R, et al. The importance of the feasibility study: lessons from a study of the hand-held fan used to relieve dyspnea in people who are breathless at rest. Palliat Med 2016;30(5):504–9.
16. Long term domiciliary oxygen therapy in chronic hypoxic cor pulmonale complicating chronic bronchitis and emphysema. Report of the Medical Research Council Working Party. Lancet 1981;1(8222):681–6.
17. Continuous or nocturnal oxygen therapy in hypoxemic chronic obstructive lung disease: a clinical trial. Nocturnal Oxygen Therapy Trial Group. Ann Intern Med 1980;933:391–8.
18. Stoller J, Panos J, Krachman S, et al. Oxygen therapy for patients with COPD: current evidence and the long-term oxygen treatment trial. Chest 2010;138(1):179–87.
19. Drummond MB, Blackford AL, Benditt JO, et al, NETT Investigators. Continuous oxygen use in nonhypoxemic emphysema patients identifies a high-risk subset of patients: retrospective analysis of the National Emphysema Treatment Trial. Chest 2008;1343:497–506.
20. Nonoyama ML, Brooks D, Lacasse Y, et al. Oxygen therapy during exercise training in chronic obstructive pulmonary disease. Cochrane Database Syst Rev 2007;(2):CD005372.
21. Guyatt GH, McKim DA, Austin P, et al. Appropriateness of domiciliary oxygen delivery. Chest 2000;118:1303–8.
22. Ben-Aharon I, Grafter-Gvili A, Leibovici L, et al. Interventions for alleviating cancer-related dyspnea: a systemic review and meta-analysis. Acta Oncol 2012;51:996–1008.
23. Abernethy A, McDonald C, Frith P, et al. Effect of palliative oxygen versus room air in relief of breathlessness in patients with refractory dyspnoea: a double-blind, randomized controlled trial. Lancet 2010;376:784–93.
24. Johnson M, Abernethy A, Currow D. The evidence base for oxygen for chronic refractory breathlessness: issues, gaps, and a future work plan. J Pain Symptom Manage 2013;45(4):763–75.
25. Mularski RA, Campbell ML, Asch SM, et al. A review of quality of care evaluation for the palliation of dyspnea. Am J Respir Crit Care Med 2010;181(6):534–8.
26. Campbell ML, Templin T, Walch J. A respiratory distress observation scale for patients unable to self-report dyspnea. J Palliat Med 2010;13(3):285–90.
27. Campbell M, Yarandi H, Dove-Meadows E. Oxygen is nonbeneficial for most patients who are near death. J Pain Symptom Manage 2013;45(3):517–23.

The Role of Intravenous Fluids and Enteral or Parenteral Nutrition in Patients with Life-limiting Illness

Meghan E. Lembeck, MD[a], Colette R. Pameijer, MD[b], Amy M. Westcott, MD[c],*

KEYWORDS

- Artificial hydration • Artificial nutrition • Intravenous fluids • Life-limiting illness
- Dying • End of life

KEY POINTS

- Discuss the risks and benefits of artificial nutrition or hydration in life-limiting illness with the patient and the family and/or decision maker.
- Describe artificial nutrition and hydration as a medical intervention.
- Explain the principles of comfort feeding and present this as an option.
- Families and decision makers often carry end-of-life decisions with them after their loved one dies.

INTRODUCTION

The inability to feed or hydrate a patient is an increasingly common consequence of both benign and malignant conditions. Patients and families are often asked their preference for artificial nutrition or hydration (ANH) in life-limiting situations, but there is little information to guide this decision making, especially related to cost-effective care. ANH is considered a medical intervention, and therefore carries some degree of invasiveness (ie, intravenous [IV] access) and risk for complication (ie, infection). ANH is not beneficial for patients with end-stage dementia[1] and 3 major organizations have highlighted this in the Choosing Wisely campaign.[2] However, there are situations, such as head and neck cancers, cerebrovascular accident, amyotrophic lateral

Disclosure: The authors have nothing to disclose.
[a] Internal Medicine, PinnacleHealth Primary Care, Annville Family Medicine, 475 North Weaber Street, Annville, PA 17003, USA; [b] Penn State College of Medicine, 500 University Drive, Mail Code H149, PO Box 850, Hershey, PA 17033, USA; [c] Geriatric and Palliative Medicine, Penn State College of Medicine, 500 University Drive, Mail Code H106, PO Box 850, Hershey, PA 17033, USA
* Corresponding author.
E-mail address: awestcott@hmc.psu.edu

Med Clin N Am 100 (2016) 1131–1141
http://dx.doi.org/10.1016/j.mcna.2016.04.019
0025-7125/16/$ – see front matter © 2016 Elsevier Inc. All rights reserved.

sclerosis, human immunodeficiency virus and acquired immunodeficiency syndrome, and cystic fibrosis, in which patients benefit from ANH. However, there are cases in which the burdens of ANH outweigh the benefits and possibly prolong the patient's suffering. Each patient and family may have different expectations for ANH. It is important to first outline what both hope to achieve with ANH. There are instances of people wishing to focus on quality of life and others in which the focus is on quantity. The reality is that most people wish to focus on both. This article cover 3 specific scenarios, including dementia, malignancy, and actively dying, in the hope of highlighting the best approach to ANH in patients with life-limiting illness.

EVALUATION OF PATIENTS FOR USE OF ARTIFICIAL NUTRITION OR HYDRATION

The evaluation of a patient for ANH or parenteral nutrition (PN) should include consideration of the following:

- Patient and/or family goals of care. These should include a discussion of what interventions are acceptable (additional tubes or lines), who is going to administer the support (family, visiting nurse, nursing home staff), and the practicalities of these support measures (tube feeds or PN require being attached to a pump and IV pole, blood work may be involved to monitor electrolyte levels). Although these support measures sound appealing at first, the implementation can be intrusive to the patient and family, and may isolate the patient by restricting activity and/or social interactions.
- Physiologic assessment. Percentage weight loss; electrolyte abnormalities; nutritional status reflected by albumin, prealbumin, or transferrin levels; and fluid balance to include gastrointestinal (GI) losses.
  - ○ Cachexia is a complex clinical syndrome of malnutrition and weight loss associated with advanced stages of various diseases. Cachexia in patients with neurologic disease is physiologically different from cachexia in patients with cancer, despite the end result seeming similar. In both situations, patients need to be carefully monitored for the effects of nutritional support, to avoid refeeding syndrome or overfeeding. Electrolyte imbalance, including hypokalemia, hypophosphatemia, and hypomagnesemia, is a hallmark of refeeding syndrome. However, cachexia associated with cancer is typically refractory to intervention, with rare gains in any measurable parameter such as weight, quality of life, or survival.[3]
- Access for nutritional support. Is the GI tract functional? What tubes or lines does the patient have already? The GI tract is always the preferred approach for supporting a patient.
- Anticipated duration of support.
- Reassessment. Once an intervention has been implemented, the patient should be assessed regularly for benefits, possible side effects, and tolerance of the intervention. Clinicians should gauge continued acceptance of the intervention and any change in patient or family goals.
- Consideration of other factors that affect a patient's ability or desire to eat are discussed later.

SETTING THE STAGE FOR THE DISCUSSION: 2 CASES
Case 1: A Case of Advanced Dementia

In the case of advanced dementia, the patient's decline has usually been progressive over years. There is an expectation by the general public that memory will slowly fade away, but it may be even more distressing to watch a loved one lose the ability to perform the activities of daily living (ADLs) that are often taken for granted. For example, the patient's disease may advance such that the patient is no longer able to eat unassisted. The patient may also develop dysphagia, predisposing to complications such as severe malnutrition, impaired healing, and recurrent aspiration pneumonia. When these complications occur, the patient's caregiver may be required to make a decision between moving forward with ANH or attempting to improve oral intake with assisted feedings. Ultimately, the basis for this decision comes down to the goals of care that have been determined by the patient and the family.

The case of SW helps to show the process of making such a decision. She is a 78-year-old woman who was diagnosed with Alzheimer dementia 6 years ago. She is currently nonverbal, unable to follow commands, and requires assistance with all ADLs. She is a resident in the dementia unit of a nursing home and is being evaluated today by the facility's physician. SW's daughter, M, who is her surrogate decision maker, is at the bedside. SW has recently been having difficulty swallowing, is losing weight, has a stage II sacral pressure ulcer, and has been hospitalized twice in the past 4 months for aspiration pneumonia. M is concerned about her mother's nutrition and her risk for continued aspiration. She would like to learn more about the different options for nutrition and asks whether a feeding tube can be placed temporarily to improve SW's intake and prevent aspiration.

Case 2: A Case of Malignancy

A final common pathway of many GI malignancies involves advanced intra-abdominal disease with bowel dysfunction and/or mechanical obstruction. A minority of these bowel obstructions may be focal, and may be managed with stents, surgical resection, or bypass (including a stoma). However, it is more common for obstruction to be multi-level, and survival is usually measured in weeks. The nausea and bloating associated with bowel obstruction can usually be managed pharmacologically, but the inability to eat can be distressing for the patient and the caregivers.

Consider the case of KR, a 60-year-old woman with peritoneal carcinomatosis from appendiceal cancer. She has progressive disease, is not tolerating chemotherapy, and has no therapeutic surgical options. She has decreasing ability to tolerate oral intake, with associated nausea and bloating. The patient and family expressed the goal of trying another chemotherapy agent, which she would only receive if she was able to tolerate a diet. She was managed with octreotide and a low-residue diet, with resolution of her symptoms. ANH was not necessary at this time. Her symptoms eventually returned, with frequent episodes of vomiting. A discussion regarding whether or not to place a percutaneous endoscopic gastrostomy (PEG) tube became necessary.

OPTIONS FOR ARTIFICIAL NUTRITION OR HYDRATION
Total Enteral Nutrition

Total enteral nutrition (TEN) is a form of artificial nutrition used when a patient is no longer able to meet nutritional requirements with oral intake alone, and the GI tract is able to be used. Long-term artificial nutrition (>4 weeks) is most often administered through a surgically placed PEG tube or, less commonly, a percutaneous endoscopic jejunostomy (PEJ) tube.

In cases of life-limiting illness, the goals that are commonly stated by patients and families when considering placement of a feeding tube and the start of TEN include the following:

- To decrease the risk of aspiration pneumonia
- To improve nutritional status

- To decrease the risk of developing pressure ulcers
- To improve functional status and quality of life
- To increase survival

However, there is no evidence to support these goals as benefits of TEN, and some may be worsened by placement of a PEG tube. For instance, PEG tubes do not prevent the aspiration of oral secretions or regurgitated gastric material. A 1996 review of articles including patients with neurogenic dysphagia concluded that there is some evidence that the risk of aspiration pneumonia increases with tube feedings.[4] Based on their findings, the investigators recommended manual feeding for most conscious patients. A 1992 study by Kadakia and colleagues[5] concluded that, "aspiration is not prevented by PEJ, continues to be a major problem after PEJ, and becomes manifest for the first time after PEG."

Pressure ulcers confer significant morbidity in any patient with a terminal diagnosis. A 2012 study by Teno and colleagues[6] using the Minimum Data Set, concluded that not only were pressure ulcers in nursing home residents with PEG tubes less likely to heal than in those without PEG tubes but PEG tube use seemed to be associated with an increased risk of the development of new pressure ulcers because of decreased mobility.

Perhaps one of the most counterintuitive conclusions is that neither nutritional nor functional status is improved by tube feeding. In a 1992 study by Henderson and colleagues,[7] chronically ill patients continued to lose weight even when the tube feeds were composed of adequate calories. Kaw and Sekas[8] determined in 1994 that there was no improvement in functional status after the placement of a PEG tube. It is likely that the underlying disease that leads to a patient being eligible for tube feeds is advanced, and simply increasing intake does not change the overall trajectory of the disease.

In a review by Sampson and colleagues[9] from the Cochrane Database in 2009, the investigators evaluated evidence of the benefits and risks of TEN in advanced dementia. There were no randomized controlled trials available, but 7 observational controlled studies were included. The investigators concluded that there was no evidence to support benefits of TEN in advanced dementia and a lack of data outlining the adverse effects.

Aside from the lack of evidence to support these commonly held beliefs, there is a great deal of behavioral morbidity associated with the use of PEG tubes. Consider that residents in nursing homes receiving tube feeds no longer receive meals in the dining hall, where they may benefit from social interactions with other residents. Instead, they are confined to their rooms, connected to machines. They also no longer have the opportunity to experience the pleasure of taste, which is a measure of the quality of life for many. Furthermore, patients with advanced dementia who have PEG tubes do not understand the principle behind the tubes protruding from their bodies, and may attempt to rid themselves of the unfamiliar apparatus, creating the potential for harm when pulling at the tube and the consideration of the use of physical restraints.

Regarding nutrition in patients with advanced dementia, multiple professional medical organizations, including the Society for Post-Acute and Long-Term Care Medicine, the American Academy of Hospice and Palliative Medicine, and the American Geriatrics Society, all recommend against the insertion of percutaneous feeding tubes, with oral assisted feedings supported as the preferred method.[2] Despite this recommendation and evidence that a percutaneous feeding tube does not meet commonly stated goals of care as outlined earlier, many patients and families are choosing artificial nutrition in terminal, life-limiting illness. Mitchell and colleagues[10] performed a cross-sectional study of 186,835 patients with advanced cognitive impairment who were residents in Medicare or Medicaid-certified US nursing homes in 1999, and found that 34% of these subjects had feeding tubes. In a follow-up study in 2002, Teno and colleagues[11] reported that the rate of nursing home residents with severe cognitive impairment with a feeding tube ranged from 3.8% to 44.8%.

Parenteral Nutrition

PN remains a controversial option in end-of-life care. Most oncologic physicians in the United States do not recommend PN, because it is thought to prolong the patient's suffering. Mercadante and colleagues[12] reviewed the use of PN in an acute palliative care unit in Italy over an 18-month time frame, and found only 10 patients in 750 admissions who were receiving PN. Four patients started PN during the admission. One month after discharge from the unit only 2 patients remained on PN, with the others having died or had stopped the PN. The most common indication for PN was bowel obstruction or dysphagia. As with hydration, there are few data to guide decisions about PN. A recent Cochrane Review found no randomized trials, and only 5 prospective, uncontrolled trials on nutrition in palliative care, and no recommendations for practice were deemed possible.[13] However, on closer review of these studies there were some trends that should be noted. Three of the studies involved patients with advanced cancer receiving PN, whereas the others involved nonmalignant disease and enteral feeding. The studies of PN and advanced cancer were overall favorable, with investigators reporting benefits such as improved energy and the psychological benefit of nutritional support.[14,15] Chermesh and colleagues[16] did find higher rates of PN-related complications in patients with malignancy compared with a control group receiving PN for nonmalignant disease, with 25% of patients having a complication. In all 3 studies, patients received PN for at least 2 weeks, and commonly for several months.

The American Society for Parenteral and Enteral Nutrition does not address the subject of PN at the end of life, but the European Society for Clinical Nutrition and Metabolism does address this issue. The European guidelines suggest offering PN if a patient's enteral nutrition is insufficient, the expected survival is more than 2 to 3 months, the PN can be expected to stabilize or improve performance status or quality of life, and the patient desires this method of nutritional support.[14] Missing from the guidelines are recommendations for the consideration of stopping PN.

A significant challenge for both starting and stopping PN is estimating a patient's survival time. It is estimated that death from starvation will occur in 1 month, or perhaps sooner in a patient with advanced cancer. It may be difficult to determine whether a patient dies from disease or starvation and the ethics of PN in this setting can be argued. It may be unethical to allow a patient to die of starvation, but it may also be unethical to prolong a patient's suffering. The question of suffering is subjective, and the suffering may or may not be related to starvation. This brings clinicians no closer to any guidelines, except to say that PN may be appropriate for patients with poor GI function and an estimated survival time of at least 1 month, with the understanding that there will come a time when the PN should be discontinued. A clear discussion with the patient and family before starting PN is paramount, with the identification of goals of therapy and anticipated stopping points.

BRINGING IT ALL TOGETHER: REVISITING THE CASES
Case 1: A Case of Advanced Dementia

SW's physician discusses options for TEN and alternatives to ANH with SW and her daughter, M. The physician assesses the goals of care for SW by asking M what was important to SW in her life. They discuss her love of reading, needlepoint, and listening to opera. M says that of those three, her mother is only able to listen to opera in her current functional state, and that this seems to calm her down when she is agitated. M tells the physician that her mother had always been a very independent woman, who would never want to be bound to a bed and would not want any permanent tubes. The physician assesses M's understanding of the natural course of dementia, and finds that she recognizes that the disease is progressive and in its terminal stages, but that she did not consider the irreversibility of SW's swallowing difficulty. The physician further clarifies the following regarding the feeding tube:

- It would be a permanent intervention in this terminal stage
- It does not prevent oral secretion aspiration
- It is unlikely to result in significant improvement in nutritional or functional status
- It does not promote healing of pressure ulcers

The physician offers oral assisted feeding for taste and comfort as an alternative option. On careful consideration, M notes that a feeding tube would not be consistent with her mother's goals, and a decision is made to focus on comfort without invasive interventions.

Case 2: A Case of Malignancy

Recall the case of KR, the 60-year-old woman with peritoneal carcinomatosis from appendiceal cancer. On further discussion with the patient, her physician learned that the vomiting was very distressing for KR and her family, and that she still desired to eat food. A PEG tube was placed to decompress her stomach as needed. Initially the PEG tube output was low enough that she could still stay hydrated with oral intake, thus ANH initially was not necessary. The PEG tube provided effective palliation for several weeks, until she progressed again and vomited despite the PEG tube being open to gravity continuously. During this hospitalization, she developed significant hypokalemia and dehydration caused by the volume of gastric drainage, and she received IV fluids and potassium. She was discharged home with daily IV fluids, although she developed peripheral edema and shortness of breath. She requested that the IV fluids be discontinued. Her condition declined quickly and she entered hospice care, dying 6 weeks later.

KR's decline in oral intake occurred over several months. Although the patient's family was very concerned about her poor intake, the patient herself only complained about the vomiting and fatigue, with less interest in food. ANH in this situation could have been considered at several points in time:

- Her initial presentation
- At the time of PEG tube placement
- Progression of her obstruction/dysfunction

In the acute care setting clinicians may replace gastric drainage in a 1:1 or 0.5:1 ratio, to avoid dehydration and metabolic alkalosis. However, the few data that exist about ANH at the end of life suggest that there is no physiologic benefit, although there may be psychological benefit for the patient and caregivers. Because decisions about ANH incorporate personal and religious beliefs, cultural norms, and patient age,[17] many clinicians think that if there are strong spiritual or religious beliefs behind the psychological benefit then it is justified. In the setting of chronic and irreversible bowel obstruction, the use of ANH should be considered carefully, because the additional risk of fluid overload and bowel edema may outweigh any benefit. A survey of adult patients with advanced cancer and their caregivers found that older patients were more likely to decline ANH, and caregivers of older patients also were more likely to decline ANH for the patient. The survey also found that caregivers were more concerned with the physical symptoms of hunger, thirst, or pain than the patients; patients were more bothered by discussion of ANH than their families.[17]

BARRIERS TO NOT PROVIDING ARTIFICIAL NUTRITION OR HYDRATION
The Do-something Mindset

In this age of major advances in medicine and technology, with real gains in quantity of life, it is often difficult for patients, families, and even physicians to accept that there may be nothing to offer to address these concerns. This situation leads to multiple interventions, such as placing a feeding tube, in the last days and weeks of life with questionable benefit, potential complications, and significant cost. Palecek and colleagues[18] provided some insight into the reasoning behind the decision to place a percutaneous feeding tube in a patient with terminal dementia. They postulate that this may partially be caused by the language used. Often, not using ANH can be wrongly interpreted as a decision not to feed. The implication of doing nothing is a powerfully uncomfortable prospect, albeit an inaccurate interpretation. In contrast, the do-everything mindset is a reassuring standard, although frequently out of alignment with the patient's goals of care. Furthermore, there is often a fear that the patient will suffer because of hunger and thirst. McCann and colleagues[19] performed a prospective evaluation of 32 cognitively intact patients with terminal illness in a comfort care unit and showed that two-thirds of the patients never reported feeling hungry and 11 only reported these symptoms during the first quarter of their stay. The investigators note that some of these patients even "experienced abdominal discomfort and nausea when they ate to please their families."[19] Palecek and colleagues[18] proposed a comfort-feeding-only order set that is personalized to each patient. This order is assisted oral feedings by caregivers that allows a greater focus on comfort and personal interaction and is therefore in stark contrast with the idea of doing nothing.

Regulatory Considerations

Fincune and colleagues[20] argued that the use of tube feedings might lead to the perception by regulatory bodies that nursing homes are providing adequate nutrition. As such, they could potentially avoid sanctions for negligence based on resident weight loss, minimize bad publicity, and reduce the risk of litigation for the nursing home. The United States Government Accountability Office released a report to congressional requesters in 2008[21] regarding state monitoring of nursing homes, with the conclusion that state surveyors were missing serious deficiencies underlying poor quality of care. One of these deficiencies was identified as untreated weight loss. The 2004 State Operations Manual[22] for guidance to surveyors of long-term care facilities states that one criterion for significant change in a resident's physical condition is the "emergence of an unplanned weight loss problem (5% change in 30 days or 10% change in 180 days)." Although attempts are made throughout the manual to support "individualized interventions" and "resident choice," vague statements such as "continuing weight loss...despite reasonable efforts," places nursing home administrators in the difficult position of acting as interpreters of how "reasonable effort" is defined. Once again, this could support the concept that "doing something" is better than the inappropriately perceived "doing nothing."

Financial Considerations

For residents in nursing homes with advanced dementia, clinicians must consider the comparative costs of caring for a resident with a feeding tube versus one who is receiving manual assistance for comfort feeding. Mitchell and colleagues[23] determined that the cost in time dedicated to each resident by staff was greater for those receiving assisted feeding than for those who were tube fed, thereby incurring a greater financial cost. Daily cost was estimated at $4219 ± $1546 for care of residents with assisted feeding (N = 11), versus $2379 ± $1032 for care of residents with tube feeding (N = 11; P value = .006). Perhaps even more significant is the comparison of time spent on feeding activities by nursing staff, totaling 25.2 minutes ± 12.9 minutes for those with feeding tubes, versus 72.8 minutes ± 16.5 minutes for those receiving assisted feeding. In addition, the overall reimbursement from Medicaid was greater for the tube-fed cohort in at least 26 states. This finding was partially accounted for by the initial cost of tube placement and emergency department visits for complications related to the tube feeding, both of which are usually covered by Medicare. The combination of these two factors could represent a financial incentive to promote tube feeding, in general, for residents of nursing care facilities with nutritional deficiencies and weight loss.

Extended care facilities are not the only agencies of health systems that stand to benefit financially from tube feeding. Specialists who place the feeding tube clearly benefit from monetary compensation, and hospitals may benefit by maximizing bed management when nursing care facilities are more willing to accept residents who are tube fed. It costs roughly $1000 for each placement of a feeding tube,[24] and new feeding tubes often qualify for skilled days in a nursing home. A change to the reimbursement practices for these facilities may help to promote medical decision making based on evidence. In addition, the education of patients, families, and health care professionals; modification of federal regulations for nursing homes; and reform of the litigation landscape may reduce incentives that influence these decisions.[20]

Lack of Health Care Provider Education

When 500 primary care physicians were surveyed by Shega and colleagues,[25] most of those who completed their questionnaire had inaccurate perceptions that caused them to overestimate the benefit of placing a feeding tube. The most impressive results from this study concluded that more than 75% of physicians thought that PEG tubes decreased the risk of aspiration pneumonia, more than 90% thought that TEN in advanced dementia improves nutritional status, and most of the participants thought that tube feeding decreased the risk of pressure ulcers. This finding clearly shows that additional education is required among health care providers.

METHODS FOR ENCOURAGING ORAL FEEDING
Oral Assisted Comfort Feeding

Assisted oral feeding is a technique used for palliative purposes in terminal illness, when adequate nutrition is no longer a goal of care. This technique is used for the patient's comfort and has several benefits. It allows patients to sit at a table with others, increasing their level of social interaction and the feeling of a familiar routine, which is especially important in patients with a diagnosis of dementia.[26] It also provides an opportunity for caregivers and family members to bond with the patients during this one-on-one time, increasing the level of communication and engagement. From a comfort standpoint, the patients are able to stimulate the sense of taste, which is frequently listed as a subjective marker for quality of life.

Discontinuation of Nonessential Medications

Patients with terminal illness often are on multiple medications. Adverse effects of these medications can interfere with the patients' eating patterns. Therefore, frequent reevaluation of each medication to assess benefits and risks is essential. Some of the most common examples include the following:

- Anticholinergics leading to xerostomia
- Sedatives causing social withdrawal and decreased attention
- Oral bisphosphonates resulting in reflux symptoms and dysphagia
- Nonsteroidal antiinflammatory drugs causing abdominal discomfort and anorexia

Therapeutic Management of Swallowing Disorders

Swallowing disorders commonly occur in malignancy, stroke, and progressive neurologic diseases. Some of the signs can be distressing to patients and families. The patient may be observed to choke or cough while eating or have repeated episodes of emesis or regurgitation. In other instances, aspiration of solids and liquids may go unnoticed. Repeated episodes can lead to recurrent aspiration pneumonias, poor appetite, or weight loss caused by food avoidance. If a swallowing disorder is suspected, a reasonable next step is to have a full speech and swallow evaluation. This evaluation could allow an individualized plan to be determined for each patient. The elements of such a plan could include body repositioning and/or a change in the texture of solids (ie, pureed) and liquids (with use of thickeners).

Dental and Oral Care

Oral hygiene should be consistently evaluated in terminally ill patients. Appropriate fit of dentures and regular use of those dentures should be ensured. Oral lesions that could lead to impaired mastication should also be evaluated on a regular basis. Artificial saliva can also be used in patients with xerostomia to improve mouth dryness, taste alteration, and chewing difficulties.[27]

A SPECIAL CASE: WHEN A PATIENT IS ACTIVELY DYING

As was the case with both of the patients described earlier, as patients enter into their final days, hydration is often a concern. Guidelines set out by Blinderman and Billings[28] for comfort care in dying patients include to "Encourage oral assisted eating for pleasure but respectfully inform patients and families that the administration of intravenous fluids and nutrition through a feeding tube has no benefit in terms of comfort or survival at this phase of illness."[28] **Table 1** provides a side-by-side benefit-versus-burden analysis. Final days are described as when a patient starts actively dying, with signs such as no longer taking any food by mouth, terminal secretions, Cheyne-Stokes breathing, and mottling of extremities. Families are concerned that their loved ones will starve to death. Providing ongoing education about the death and dying process is important to minimize the suffering of both patients and families.

Table 1	
Actively dying patients: benefits versus burdens of IV fluids	
Benefit	**Burden**
Address patient/family preferences	Increase secretions
Address spiritual/religious preferences	Edema/anasarca
Prevent dehydration	Loose stool

Discussing the potential side effects of providing fluids once someone is actively dying, such as worsening of secretions and edema, often dissuades families from this intervention. Some families may need a trial of fluids for a specific amount (eg, 1 L) or period of time (eg, 1 day) to see whether there is any benefit to the patient. It is important for health care providers to be honest about what that benefit might be but also to support families through the process. Also, special circumstances exist around the need to provide ANH for spiritual or religious reasons.

SUMMARY

Many health care providers, patients, and families struggle with weighing the benefits and burdens of ANH. It is important to consider patient and family goals of care, quality of life, and risks related to ANH. There are alternative approaches, such as comfort feeding, correcting reversible issues, and/or a trial of ANH, which may be of more value to patients and families living with life-limiting illnesses. A patient-centered and family-centered approach, along with the education of all those involved in providing end-of-life care, helps to provide high-quality and cost-effective measures for patients in the terminal stages of their lives.

REFERENCES

1. Teno JM, Gozalo PL, Mitchell SL, et al. Does feeding tube insertion and its timing improve survival? J Am Geriatr Soc 2012;60(10):1918–21.
2. American Board of Internal Medicine Foundation. Available at: http://www.choosingwisely.org/. Accessed December 22, 2015.
3. Palesty JA, Dudrick SJ. Cachexia, malnutrition, the refeeding syndrome, and lessons from Goldilocks. Surg Clin North Am 2011;91(3):653–73.
4. Finucane TE, Bynum JP. Use of tube feeding to prevent aspiration pneumonia. Lancet 1996;348(9039):1421–4.
5. Kadakia SC, Sullivan HO, Starnes E. Percutaneous endoscopic gastrostomy or jejunostomy and the incidence of aspiration in 79 patients. Am J Surg 1992;164(2):114–8.
6. Teno JM, Gozalo P, Mitchell SL, et al. Feeding tubes and the prevention or healing of pressure ulcers. Arch Intern Med 2012;172(9):697–701.
7. Henderson CT, Trumbore LS, Mobarhan S, et al. Prolonged tube feeding in long-term care: nutritional status and clinical outcomes. J Am Coll Nutr 1992;11(3):309–25.
8. Kaw M, Sekas G. Long-term follow-up of consequences of percutaneous endoscopic gastrostomy (PEG) tubes in nursing home patients. Dig Dis Sci 1994;39(4):738–43.
9. Sampson EL, Candy B, Jones L. Enteral tube feeding for older people with advanced dementia. Cochrane Database Syst Rev 2009;(2):CD007209.
10. Mitchell SL, Teno JM, Roy J, et al. Clinical and organizational factors associated with feeding tube use among nursing home residents with advanced cognitive impairment. JAMA 2003;290(1):73–80.
11. Teno JM, Mor V, DeSilva D, et al. Use of feeding tubes in nursing home residents with severe cognitive impairment. JAMA 2002;287(24):3211–2.
12. Mercadante S, Caruselli A, Villari P, et al. Frequency and indications of parenteral nutrition in an acute palliative care unit. Nutr Cancer 2015;67(6):1010–3.
13. Good P, Richard R, Syrmis W, et al. Medically assisted nutrition for adult palliative care patients. Cochrane Database Syst Rev 2014;(4):CD006274.

14. Bozzetti F, Arends J, Lundholm K, et al. ESPEN Guidelines on Parenteral Nutrition: non-surgical oncology. Clin Nutr 2009;28(4):445–54.
15. Orrevall Y, Tishelman C, Permert J. Home parenteral nutrition: a qualitative interview study of the experiences of advanced cancer patients and their families. Clin Nutr 2005;24(6):961–70.
16. Chermesh I, Mashiach T, Amit A, et al. Home parenteral nutrition (HTPN) for incurable patients with cancer with gastrointestinal obstruction: do the benefits outweigh the risks? Med Oncol 2011;28(1):83–8.
17. Bukki J, Unterpaul T, Nubling G, et al. Decision making at the end of life–cancer patients' and their caregivers' views on artificial nutrition and hydration. Support Care Cancer 2014;22(12):3287–99.
18. Palecek EJ, Teno JM, Casarett DJ, et al. Comfort feeding only: a proposal to bring clarity to decision-making regarding difficulty with eating for persons with advanced dementia. J Am Geriatr Soc 2010;58(3):580–4.
19. McCann RM, Hall WJ, Groth-Juncker A. Comfort care for terminally ill patients. The appropriate use of nutrition and hydration. JAMA 1994;272(16):1263–6.
20. Finucane TE, Christmas C, Leff BA. Tube feeding in dementia: how incentives undermine health care quality and patient safety. J Am Med Dir Assoc 2007; 8(4):205–8.
21. Office USGA. Report to congressional requesters: nursing homes federal monitoring surveys demonstrate continued understatement of serious care problems and CMS oversight weaknesses. 2008.
22. Centers for Medicare & Medicaid Services. State operations manual appendix PP: guidance to surveyors for long term care facilities. 2004.
23. Mitchell SL, Buchanan JL, Littlehale S, et al. Tube-feeding versus hand-feeding nursing home residents with advanced dementia: a cost comparison. J Am Med Dir Assoc 2003;4(1):27–33.
24. Boston Scientific. Guidepoint reimbursement resources: 2015 coding & payment quick reference select enteral feeding procedures. 2015.
25. Shega JW, Hougham GW, Stocking CB, et al. Barriers to limiting the practice of feeding tube placement in advanced dementia. J Palliat Med 2003;6(6):885–93.
26. Hanson L, Ersek M, Gilliam R, et al. Oral feeding options for people with dementia: a systematic review. J Am Geriatr Soc 2011;59(3):463–72.
27. Salom M, Hachulla E, Bertolus C, et al. Efficacy and safety of a new oral saliva equivalent in the management of xerostomia: a national, multicenter, randomized study. Oral Surg Oral Med Oral Pathol Oral Radiol 2015;119(3):301–9.
28. Blinderman C, Billings J. Comfort care for patients dying in the hospital. N Engl J Med 2015;373:2549–61.

Index

Note: Page numbers of article titles are in **boldface** type.

A

Med Clin N Am 100 (2016) 1143–1155
http://dx.doi.org/10.1016/S0025-7125(16)37313-8
0025-7125/16/$ – see front matter

medical.theclinics.com

Moving?

Make sure your subscription moves with you!

To notify us of your new address, find your **Clinics Account Number** (located on your mailing label above your name), and contact customer service at:

Email: journalscustomerservice-usa@elsevier.com

800-654-2452 (subscribers in the U.S. & Canada)
314-447-8871 (subscribers outside of the U.S. & Canada)

Fax number: 314-447-8029

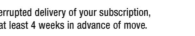

Elsevier Health Sciences Division
Subscription Customer Service
3251 Riverport Lane
Maryland Heights, MO 63043

*To ensure uninterrupted delivery of your subscription, please notify us at least 4 weeks in advance of move.

Printed and bound by CPI Group (UK) Ltd, Croydon, CR0 4YY

03/10/2024

01040390-0019